This book is fo

You have ever, ever said,

'No dessert for me, thanks. Am really full!'

'Why do the dress sizes vary from shop to shop? I'm a 14 in Next!'

'I've just started running'

'I think it's my thyroid, as I never eat anything!'

'I can't get this dress on over my head! My ears really hurt'

'I will start my diet on Monday'

'My husband says my stomach is like a pair of buttocks'

'At least if I get cancer, I have some reserves to fall back on'

'Are crisps one of my five a day?'

'How much do contact lenses weigh?'

'The camera adds two stone'

'When did Mars Bars get smaller?'

'I wonder if my tonsils are fat?'

Midway up a flight of stairs, 'Just spotted some fluff. Won't be too long'

'At least when I die, I'll be a skeleton.' To which your best friend replies disloyally, 'E-ven-tually'

WHAT PEOPLE HAVE SAID ABOUT LIZ JONES

'A better writer than Helen Fielding'
The Evening Standard

'The best comic creation since Alan Partridge'
Lynn Barber,
The Sunday Times Magazine

'The Tracey Emin of literature'
The Observer

'The Queen of Confessional Journalism'
BBC Radio 4

I absolutely loved this book! I cannot rave about it enough. This was the type of book that I read in record time as I couldn't put it down. It was hilarious, witty and some parts made me absolutely laugh out loud at them. I think anyone that has struggled

with weight issues should especially read this book, as so much you just nod your head at and makes you think 'wow I am not the only one that thought that' it also has a powerful message to it and it will be one that I will re-read again and again.
Rose Shepherd Saga Magazine

Wonderfully witty and painfully honest - I couldn't stop reading."
Deborah Ross, The Times;

"Liz Jones is a fearless, funny truth-teller about the female condition. 8 and a half stone will bring comfort and joy to fans of her column and to anyone who ever removed their contact lenses to weigh less as they step on those tyrannical scales."

Allison Pearson, The Telegraph

ACKNOWLEDGMENTS

Susan Mears
Mike French
Nicola Bebb
Nirpal Dhaliwal
Dawn Bartlett
Chris Davis
Derrick Gask
Helen Saxty
Sue Needleman
Sue Peart
Ted Verity

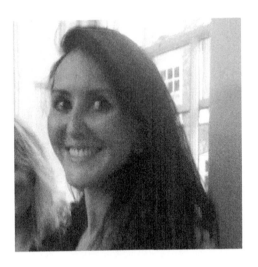

ABOUT LIZ JONES

Liz Jones, former editor-in-chief of Marie Claire – where she ran a high-profile campaign to ban skinny models – fashion editor at the Daily Mail and now columnist at the Mail on Sunday …

Liz grew up in Essex and suffered from anorexia from the age of 11 until her late thirties and, well, now a bit really.

The most shared, most commented on writer on MailOnline for ten years, with 69 million readers across the world.

Shortlisted five times in the last six years as Columnist of the Year at the British Press Awards.

Columnist of the Year 2012 at the BSME awards (or, as Liz likes to call them, the Mad Cow Bongs.)

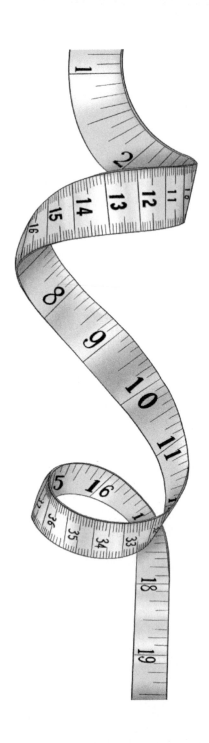

LIZ JONES

8¹/₂ STONE

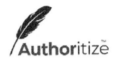

Published by
Authoritize Ltd
16, Croydon Road, Beddington,
Croydon, Surrey CR0 4PA
www.authoritize.me.uk

8 1/2 Stone by Liz Jones

ISBN 978-1-913623-55-5
© 2021 Liz Jones

Printed by 4Edge

CONTENTS

BIG PAM'S STORY

LITTLE PAM'S STORY

'A terrible beauty is born'

WB Yeats

PART 1
BIG PAM'S STORY

CHAPTER ONE
Confectionery

My top ten best sweets, in reverse order (okay, there are 13; please don't tell me I have too many sweets):

(Adopt a David Jacobs voice)

No. 13
Coffee Walnut Whip

It comes in a smart cellophane box, on a plinth, like an exhibit in a museum. The white, vanilla version is a little too sweet and synthetic looking, so cannot be good for you. The subtle coffee version, however, adds sophistication. It's a grown-up treat. How best to eat it? Nibble the walnut first, as a starter, then make a small incision in the top with any teeth you have left. Stick in tongue anteater-fashion to extract the frothy filling. Work your way round the sides in a spiral, dissolving it, before ending up with the deliciously thick disc at the bottom. Which you can suck on, a hungry piglet on a teat, for hours.

No. 12
Cadbury's Buttons

They should print on the side of the packet: little coins of happiness. These need to be always sucked, never chewed or bitten into: no one should bite chocolate; it needs to melt in the mouth. Buttons tend to stick to the roof of the mouth, tenacious as small brown fire alarms. Mum always gave me Buttons when I was off school with a sore throat or because of bullying (she felt Galaxy Counters were too sweet, and too small), and I always, always received a Buttons Easter egg, even though the teeny cellophane bag lurking inside like giblets never failed to disappoint.

No. 11
Cadbury's Flake

You can always tell a fat person by the way they eat a Flake: with a sheet tucked under each chin, a wary expression – a delicate exercise performed never in wind, and preferably indoors, in private behind a locked door. The reason for the care is in the name: Flake. It flakes, which means you could lose some of the delicious chocolate bits, which meant I always railed at the telly when the floaty model came on, eating a Flake outside, in a meadow! How on earth would you find any stray chocolate bits in a field? I mean, come on!

You know you have an overeating disorder if you abandon the Flake for a Galaxy Ripple: sealed in a bunker and guaranteed to leave no crumbs.

No. 10
Crunchie

I never eat a Crunchie for the insides, which are a bit too dusty for my liking. And I don't particularly enjoy honey. But I love a Crunchie for the chocolate. It is just so thick. It's for those days when you don't fancy a hazelnut. It's a good, solid sweet for when the baked potato just will not go soft, no matter how many times you stab it.

No. 9
Topic

The Prada of sweets, as it was always way beyond my pocket money. But boy was it worth it once you saved up doing bob-a-job: you could snuffle out the hazelnuts and enjoy the caramel. Even the red packaging is pure class, so much more festive than the dreary old monochrome Mars Bar, which doesn't make the chart as it 'has no crunch', as Mary Berry would say. A Mars Bar just sticks to the roof of your mouth, while the TV jingle – 'helps you work, rest and play' – is far too exhausting; plus I swear Mars Bars have got smaller over the years.

No. 8
Kit Kat

A regular in my school lunch box; Mum's idea of putting me on a diet was to include two 2-finger ones, in the vain hope I'd leave one foiled for the afternoon break instead of buying Smith's Crisps. That is a No. The snap is delightful, and it feels almost wholesome. I'm so glad I'd left school before they invented the Kit Kat Chunky. That would have inevitably been my new nickname, replacing Spam (it's not that I ate the luncheon meat – what a posh description for something so chavvy – but that my flesh had the same colour and texture). Kit Kats go really well with ready salted crisps: you have to eat them at the same time, though.

No. 7
Nut pyramid

It's surprising I have any teeth left, given my childhood addiction to these little towers of sugary protein. In case these have long since been banned, along with full-strength Capstan ciggies and heroin, a nut pyramid is made up of peanuts cemented together with rock-hard caramel. It will break your teeth and your willpower ALTHOUGH my theory, as I explained to Mum, is it took so much hard work to gnaw it to a stump, it actually burnt off the calories. So, a nut pyramid is really equivalent to going to the gym. Yes.

No. 6
Mint Matchmakers

The reason these knobbly little things, which come in a drawer, make the chart is because of the TV advert: it was all about being sophisticated and hosting dinner parties, and ladies dressed up to the nines, huge dining rooms echoing with tinkling laughter. You were supposed to suck on these little beauties over coffee, not inhale one on the way to school but, as a plus point, they solved the problem of what to buy Mum for Christmas for 25 years.

No. 5
A tin of Quality Street

If there is one of these tins, as big as a hippo, open in your house it must be Christmas Eve, which is always good as any diet officially ends at midnight and doesn't reconvene until January 2nd at the earliest. As an only child, there were no fights over:

The purple one: a hazelnut inside milk chocolate, surrounded by caramel, probably the biggest sweet in there, the size of my guinea pig.

The yellow toffee coin: a little bit boring, but can be sucked for hours while you wait for the turkey to be cooked all the way through.

The green triangle: hazelnut noisette, in thick milk chocolate, and a really sophisticated design. The green is just so Christmassy.

I can imagine the rivalry gets heated if you have siblings or grannies still mobile and alive, but in my house I always got first dibs, and if ever I experimented and strayed off-piste and ate something other than the three above, such as the strawberry delight in the pink wrapper – ewww! – I would just spit it out and Mum would finish it off. So, no waste there.

A small point: never, ever leave the wrappers in the tin. This is just bad manners, as it slows everyone else down by muddying the waters.

No. 4

We're quite near the top now, savouring the confectionery equivalent of a Michael Jackson or

George Michael. (And who wouldn't want to suck on them? I never guessed George was gay, by the way, despite the fingerless gloves and platinum-dipped quiff.) For me, the fourth best sweet in the world is a bar of **Cadbury's Dairy Milk WHOLENUT.**

Because eating one is taking part in a lottery: the disappointment when a chunky square is hazelnutless and barren. The joy when you get a WHOLE NUT. A moot point here, too: why make the wrapper with re-sealable edges? Why? It's almost as bad as printing on a bag of crisps: 'made for sharing' or 'family size'. You can bugger right off. Don't tell me how to eat my sweets. And 'fun size', too? I don't agree with that. Where's the fun in something so small?

No. 3
Bounty

The milk version, of course, in its baby-blue wrapper, not the plain in the red wrapper, which is disgusting. Oh, the TV advert, with its depiction of a damsel with a flower behind her ear on a tropical island, being near-drowned in surf, forced to wear a bikini, sharks circling inches away, but ecstatic because she is eating a tropical Bounty bar. Mmmmmm. I also love the fact each bullet-shaped bar comes in a little tray, as though you're about to play Scrabble. Plus, the taste of paradise. What more is there to add?

No. 2
Twix

Hmmm. Let me count the ways. First, there are two of them. Always a bonus. Second, there is biscuit, which is great if you're tired of all those hazelnuts. It fills you up, too.

It also tells a lot about you as a person. You enjoy and relish sweets, but you are not insane enough to hanker after a Wagon Wheel: way too much marshmallow, way too sickly – you will contract type 2 diabetes just by looking at a Wagon Wheel. No, a Twix is a biscuit, but a biscuit who has got married to a little piece of heaven. You can stick your Finger of Fudge. It is never enough. (Penguins were a contender for slot 2 but were disqualified for being a biscuit. It's a fine line.)

No. 1
Maltesers

It is diet, which is the reason the much loved Rolo is languishing all the way back there at No 14. Eat one of these little balls and the weight just drops off.

'Chocolates?'

'Maltesers!'

They must only come in a box, though, not a bag. A smart little box, where they roll around inside, as though in a pinball machine, drowning out all the dialogue should you be eating your Maltesers in the cinema. Again, the method of consumption must be to suck them vigorously. But they do have their drawbacks: sometimes, you will get a rogue Malteser, with a collapsed, hard and bitter honeycomb: it's as though you have just gone on a date with a really hot man who resembles David Gandy, only to discover when you get into bed that he has a penis the size of a Cheesy Wotsit.

But, on the other hand, think of the joy when you discover one last Malteser, hiding in the corner of the box, just when you thought they were all gone. A bonus Malteser. One that almost got away.

8¹/₂ STONE

CHAPTER TWO
I blame my mum

I don't eat all that stuff anymore, of course I don't. It is but a Long and Distant Memory. I'm reformed. Scared witless by all those shock reports and headlines in the papers – 'Obesity is the new smoking!' shouted one example in The Independent last week – and documentaries on TV showing only big bellies and enormous arses, accompanied by statistics on how the bigger-boned among us cost the NHS five trillion a year.

I don't eat sweets in public, anyway, in case someone reports back to my superhumanly svelte, snake-hipped husband that 'I saw her chomping on a Milky Way in Brixton Market, by the bins. I thought her jaw had been wired. Should she be sectioned? Divorced? Tasered?' I've stopped eating sweets – and doughnuts, and pizza, and white rice (it's really bad for you: the culinary equivalent of cocaine) – since I was asked at work to give, and I quote, 'the circumference of your equator' when everyone else was asked the size of their waist for my boss's stupid idea we should wear uniforms when on walkie-talkie duty at London Fashion Week. One cheeky little cow asked if I have my own moon.

But I miss those days at Brentwood High School for Girls – and, okay, last week (what can I say, I'd had a difficult end to my day when the bus driver, who must have weighed 22 stone, told me I had to swipe my Oyster card 'twice, Love', and then a First World War hero with a Zimmer frame and medals on his chest shakily offered up his seat, thinking I must be pregnant with triplets) – when dinner would involve nothing more than a visit to the psychedelic sweet counter in the corner shop on the way home from the Tube: a quick smash and grab, a flurry of foil and it was all over.

Now, though, that I'm on an 800-calorie-a-day diet, inflicted on me by my 'weight management team' (four ugly, badly dressed bastards, not one of whom can possibly weigh less than 15 stone), in a bid to stave off (starve off) type 2 diabetes (at least if I go blind I won't have to look at myself), I have to buy things with peel, and rind, and that need soaking overnight like my knickers. I have to chop these bastard things. And weigh them. I have to weigh olive oil. One teaspoon is 45 calories. Can you believe that? I have to weigh coriander and spinach. I have to read articles in magazines with titles like 'Self-care for dummies' that tell me celery juice is the new kale. Who has time to do all that when you have twins and a husband who is incapable of calling the Gas Board without mumbling 'Where's the number? Where?' And when you find the number, and give it to him, he dials it while you stand there, hands on hips, monitoring him like Hattie bleeding Jacques, and instead of telling them off he listens to their side and then says, in a tiny voice, 'That's okay. Thanks very much. Bye-bye.' Useless! How is it that men rule the world? How?

I blame the twins for my current weight gain (the nuclear warhead mushrooming, if you will): of course I do. I might have been a big bouncy baby, a chubby child, a truck-sized teen, a Tyrannosaurus early twentysomething, but at least before the twins I could fit through doors. Now, people look at me as though I'm a Chesterfield sofa that will need to come through a window, or over a Juliet balcony. It's dispiriting, to say the least. When people arrive at La Paz airport in Bolivia (I did a press trip there once, ferrying journalists to tell them about fair trade gold; I had to demonstrate and pose for photos. I think in my whole career, the most bizarre thing I have ever said was, 'Do you want me to carry on mining?') there are oxygen masks near passport control in case you pass out due to the high altitude. I need one of those outside Oxford Circus Tube. Every day feels as though I'm climbing K2 freestyle.

Absolutely everything is difficult. And I'm not just talking about the fact I have to do up my jeans with a coat hanger, prone on the carpet while the cat stands on my chest, staring intently into my eyes, headbutting me and chirruping. Or the fact thongs get sucked into crevices, never to be seen again, like a sheep who strayed into a bog on Bodmin. Or that you get wedged in revolving doors – fucking Selfridges. And turnstiles at the Tube. Or that mothers with small children look at you and shudder, and vow to dilute their child's organic apple juice to one part to every 600 of water that very night. Or that you can't cross your legs: when you try, your foot can ping, putting someone's teeth out. Or that you have to use underboob deodorant (they should draw little boobs on the TV weather map: dry, moist or why not grow cress under there?). Or that men on planes who themselves look like they're expecting triplets huff and puff and raise an eyebrow when your little meal arrives, as if you should be placed in the hold as cargo. Or that skinny women behind you at the till in Tesco, with one basket containing Pellegrino, fresh basil, Vogue and a pomegranate, say, 'Oooh, as you have a giant trolley [for which, read 'arse'], can I please go first? I have a hot date with David

Gandy to prep for.'

(I remember wheeling the twins round Sainsbury's not long after they were born and people looking at me – really badly dressed, ugly people – and then at them, then back at me, and I could see them thinking, 'Dear God. Who on earth would have sex with that? How is that even possible?')

Or that your belly button becomes infected and painful, as to clean that deep is the ablutions equivalent of fracking. Or that when you have sex (cue sound of hollow laughter), and he wants your knees over your shoulders, hands clasped round each tree trunk, your breasts upend and smother you so you turn blue, and when he occasionally opens his eyes and notices, he laughs, and says that you resemble a Smurf. 'All you need is a conical hat,' he says, dismounting, probably disappearing to wank over photos of Keira Knightley in the Chanel ad. I tell him that at least having a fat bird for a wife means he has an early-warning system as I approach (the glass of water at his side always ripples, recalling that scene in Jurassic Park), giving him time to snap his MacBook Pro shut and pretend that, for the first time in his life, he's been doing the online Sainsbury's shop but suddenly just 'needs to check the store cupboard'. Yeah, right.

He is always on about me eating 'healthily'. That gaining so much baby weight, and toddler weight, and eight-year-old weight, 'can't be good for you'. He bought me a Spiralizer for my birthday last year. And a book on how to make smoothies costing £1 from Oxfam.

But people always want you to lose weight for themselves, don't they? It can't be fun for such a young, handsome Asian man to walk into a restaurant with a blonde Essex girl who could easily be described as 'a great white'. Oh, the jibes on the mean streets of Wickford on the way home from school. 'You're going to need a bigger boat!' the lads from Brentwood Bugs would yell. 'Never heard that one before!' I countered. 'Can you not come up with anything original? I know, how about, "Fancy browsing in 250 Poundsland?"' Fucking unimaginative morons.

Oh, of course girlfriends simply love, love, LOVE you being fat, too. They can just stand beside you at the youth club disco and suddenly they're Cara Delevingne or Karlie Kloss. They are always saying things like, 'Go on, another drink won't hurt. Have a dessert! Treat yourself!' Normal-sized people, rooting around for something positive to say, usually come up with that dreaded word: bubbly. This should only be used to describe champagne. Who do they think I am, fucking eighties popstrel Sonia?

The best (okay, only) compliment anyone ever paid me at school was, 'You have really good skin.' Even today, at the grand old age of 30, I'm frequently told

'You'll age really well.' Yeah, I won't have wrinkles because everything is stretched, like a balloon. Touch any part of my body and it squeaks. With a few twists, turns and knots I could be a giraffe.

Which reminds me. There is absolutely nothing good you can say to a fat person about their size, so it's best you just don't mention it. I had a friend once – an ex-friend now, obviously – who said, apropos of nothing, 'I used to have a black cat called Squeaky. She weighed 30 kilos, which is about the size of a large Basset Hound. Her stomach would drag on the ground and go bald from the friction. The vet was outraged, but there was nothing I could do. She was just a fat cat. She used to get stuck in the cat flap and come into the lounge wearing it as a tutu, mewing for me to take it off. But the thing is, when she was 21 and got stomach cancer, and had to have chemo and could no longer eat, she had all these reserves, which really kept her going!'

Ooh, thanks for that! Really cheering. Sooo. The upshot is if I am lucky enough to get cancer and have to have chemo, at least I'm a squirrel with a secret hoard of hazelnuts buried beneath dead leaves. I will take longer to become a Gisele-like bag of bones. Life will momentarily improve. For the first time in my life, I will be ahead.

Just like every fat person in the universe, I've tried

to diet, but nothing works. The 5:2. The cabbage soup. A liquid-only diet with shakes replacing meals and a bar of sawdust for lunch. Weightwatchers. Slimming World. The carnivore diet. The Neanderthal diet. The vegan diet; sod animals, I just want to be able to varnish my own toes. Deliciously fucking Ella – privileged cunt. Fasting. The boiled egg diet. The grapefruit diet: people would ask me at school whether I was crying because I was too fat to fit inside the coloured sash for netball. 'No, no, no,' I would reassure them. 'The grapefruit got me in the eye.' Who gets attacked by breakfast? I hate myself! I have the silhouette of SpongeBob SquarePants! I'm a moving square!

The thinnest I have ever been (apart from when I was a foetus, obvs) was on the day of my wedding. I was like a Victoria's Secret model (I am sure this is how you've been picturing me, from page one), in that for the last three days before the Big Day (never was a description more apt), I didn't even take on board water. I was so dehydrated, when Neps was told to kiss the bride he got exfoliated. I was still a size 18, but at least I was able to buy a dress off-the-peg and which vaguely went in at about the halfway mark. I was so light-headed, one sip of champagne and I started hallucinating. I also rather worryingly started to rehydrate and swell up swiftly, for all the world a Vesta beef curry – imagine my thighs as the crispy noodles. I was so worried that I would relapse on the honeymoon, I secretly tried to find exotic locations that still had an Ebola outbreak; oh, for a flesh-eating disease.

Because that is what always happens after a diet. You relapse. You inflate like a hovercraft. You revert to type. You find your natural level, like Lake Victoria.

Which is why I am considering plastic surgery – after a great deal of thought and having made a list of pros and cons. Pros: I will be able to wear normal clothes, my husband might want sex with me, I might not die of a heart attack. Cons: the expense, time off work, might die. Leaps forward in technology and medical discoveries must be good for something, surely. I am thinking liposuction, and a tummy tuck to excise the strange little flap of skin that is a legacy from post-twin diet number 252. (My friend Izzy made me go to Chewton Glen in the New Forest – don't worry, it had just been refurbed – for a week, where I was on a juice-only regimen with added boot camp and wrapped in wet bandages in a bid to rearrange my organs and reduce my equator, after a particularly invasive colonic where the therapist kept finding peas: 'Mattar paneer,' I told her. 'I'm married to an Indian.') Anyway, this skin flap is currently covering my pudenda in a generous curtain, much like the one at the Royal Opera House, only not made of red velvet. I haven't told a soul yet that I'm considering going under The Knife, but I'm secretly browsing websites and imagining how great my new life will be.

Even on my 30th birthday night, when we returned from the sandwich bar at precisely 8.29 p.m., after my disastrous at-home spa and once Neps had lowered his eyes after raising them long enough to give me Harvey's Bristol Cream liqueurs in a bid to give me either liver cancer or type 2 diabetes so he can at last bury me in an extra-large grave and remarry a stick insect, I had opened my own rather ancient and heavy laptop (like mother, like daughter) and started browsing websites depicting smiling supermodels who obviously never needed to go under a knife in the first place, but were still standing there, in a red, high-cut swimsuit, boobs thrust out, back curved, one knee forward, hand on non-existent hip. This could be my birthday gift to myself, to kick off a brand-new decade: major invasive surgery and anaesthetic that might just finish me off. Browsing these sites, being taken in by the promises, is exactly the same as being addicted to Rightmove.co.uk, except instead of searching for a new house, I am looking for the perfect new body to move into: downsizing, if you will. My life will be happy, once I have a utility room, a marble wet room, an eat-in kitchen and a stomach that doesn't resemble a pair of obese buttocks. My mission, should I choose to accept it? To get down to my dream weight, a number I have not owned since I was seven.

To be eight and a half stone.

I blame my mum, really. Of course I do. Philip Larkin? You hit the nail right on the bloody head. I read somewhere (Take a Break?) that the hereditary factor for being fat is exactly the same as the hereditary factor for being tall. If your dad plays professional NBA, chances are you will always be the one selected to place the fairy on the top of the Christmas tree. If your mum is a size 22, it's very likely you will be, too.

So, my mum always had this slightly guilty look about the gills. She would grimace at the sight of me and flail herself on the back with a knotted rope when she saw me struggling with the zip of my navy skirt for school: beads of sweat would appear on my nose with the effort, even in snow. She would pen without demur a letter saying I have to be excused from swimming lessons because I have 'a virulent, incurable, highly contagious verruca that does not respond to aggressive treatment' and not tell them the truth: 'She can't even get the floral cap once owned by her gran over her big, fat head.'

But she also, rather counter-intuitively, had a Sweet Drawer. This Sweet Drawer was in the kitchen, and the Top Ten could always be found beneath the ironed tea towels – an early, completely and utterly ineffectual version of having my jaw wired shut – when I got home from school, absolutely starving, smarting from all the abuse. Occasionally, the Kit Kat would be missing, as she had eaten it with the worry of having passed on her fat genes, and also because she failed to hold onto her husband beyond my eighth birthday, also due to her fat genes. But otherwise, there it was: a rustling unlucky dip. Designed to 'keep you going till dinner time'.

I am trying to remember when I first realised that I was not quite the desired shape. (Desirable for what, I wonder now? Bikini modelling? The prima ballerina role in Swan Lake? Marathon running? Grand National jockeying? The uneven bars at the Olympics?) At primary school, I was doing pretty okay until the day we were told to put on a regulation vest and navy knickers for PE. I had never seen the legs of other little girls. Much in the same way that as a grown woman, I've never seen another woman's vagina at close hand; it took my oversexed and early seed-sowing husband to tell me that the inner and outer flaps can vary wildly and that some women have cunts like coral; the only compliment he ever paid me, aside from that 'you must be able to swim well, as your feet are like paddles', was to say overweight girls are more pleasurable to fuck, as with skinny ones there is too much knocking on the pubic bone, making him feel as though he's a waiter attempting to deliver room service.

Anyway, back to primary school, when I had never, ever seen other children naked because, as well as being an only child, Southend sea front was always too windswept to allow the removing of little floral jersey trousers as a toddler, and puffa coats, and scarves, and gloves, and woolly hats. And so it is that there I was, aged five, planted like a reluctant horse at the threshold of the gym area, gazing open-mouthed in amazement at the other little girls' unsheathed limbs. There were no rolls of fat at the top. Their legs at the bottom went in before they grew a foot. Tummies were not meant, I realised to my horror, to peek (and peak) below T-shirts in a creamy harvest moon. Arms could hang perpendicular to bodies, instead of jutting out at 45 degrees. And, oh, the indignity of being assigned a pair of plimsolls. Miss Goodwin was forced to be dispatched to the Big School, where there be Big Girls, to fetch me a pair of size 39s. I was six years old and already my age (thank you, Prince) matched my shoe size. An early epithet was 'Bungle'.

And so, from a tender age, instead of a source of fun, a confidence builder, a camaraderie maker, exercise became something I dreaded and abhorred, made excuses at all costs to avoid. My body, which until the age of six had done pretty much everything I wanted it to – play, sleep, sit (arms just long enough to cuddle one of my mum's arms, or her head), watch telly, play two-ball against the garage wall – suddenly became something to be ashamed of, a battleground, a source of abject misery and humiliation and overexposure. The enemy.

Everything got worse, of course, when I found out Mum has M&S. No, what am I thinking? MS. The signs at first that there was something wrong were subtle. She would miss putting a plate on the table, so it would crash to the floor. An arm would tingle, and not just because I was leaning in the crook of it for a story. She would be unsteady on her feet at the end of the day; she blamed the sherry, though I never saw her drink more than a thimbleful. She kept the diagnosis from me for a long time. I was a Big Girl in Big School before she finally plucked up the courage to tell me; there was no longer any way to explain away the arrival of a rail by the bath and next to the loo, or a wheelchair in the hallway, or a ramp appearing over the front step, or a woman in uniform who turned up three times a day wielding industrial-sized tubs of Sudocrem. 'Oh, she's just a friend come for coffee,' was how she explained it for ages.

Mealtimes, already a source of global conflict, with side dishes of calorie counters and charts and corsets, and smaller plates to fool the eye if not the tummy, became even more difficult. Mum now had to chop from the sitting position, which is really hard and tiring, and so of course she started to buy more ready meals: little oblongs of E numbers and salt and trans-fat that could just be slotted in the microwave after a satisfying pop, pop, pop of the cellophane. And so, while I was in high school, we both gradually grew bigger. Weight crept up on us, a stain on a shirt when someone is shot in the chest with a 12-bore shotgun. And just as deadly.

Mum started to overcompensate even more for the fact she was now confined to a wheelchair and forced to rely on benefits: and by overcompensate, I mean overfeed. I remember she would hove into view, in her wheelchair, on the edge of the playing field, to check I wasn't having a heart attack during hockey (I was always, always stuck in goal; Miss Gillett didn't even bother giving me a hockey stick, as my bulk deflected all comers), waggling a ribbon of Penguins, the worry etched on her large, Captain-Pugwash face that perhaps she should have opted for a variety pack of Clubs instead. Aged 11, I was 4 ft 11 in, and weighed 11 stone. This is the time I decided to keep a chart. It went as follows:

Monday to Friday
Breakfast
A Cox's apple: 45 cals
Half a banana: 52 cals

Lunch
A Ski yogurt, raspberry or similar: 118 cals

Dinner
Half a grilled tom: 12 cals
Grilled mushroom x 2: 30 cals
Slice of Nimble ('She's flies like a bird, etc., etc., etc.') bread: 50 cals
Can of Tab: zero cals, plus really fills you up

Total cals: 307

Saturday

The same, though I added a packet of Smiths crisps as a treat; I was really missing unfolding the little blue origami parcel of salt. That counts as exercise anyway, surely

Sunday had the added input of a roast lunch though I eschewed the Yorkshire pudding and only had one roast potato

Below this on the spread chart (aptly named, doncha think?) was my exercise regime for each day:

Sit-ups: 100 if poss, but try to get past four
Side bends: 50, easy!

Running on the spot: 10 mins, or until Mrs Cresswell next door calls Mum to complain about plaster raining on her head in her sitting room

Lunges, with hands on hip: three on each side

Squats: five (on number six, I tend to go down, but I never, ever come back up)

At the bottom of each day was a tabula rasa in which to record my weight. Over the course of 12 weeks, the projected (note that all-important P word) figure (oh, that I had a figure!) had gone from 12 stone to the magical eight and a half. It was just a matter of mathematics or, as we called it in primary school, sums. Calories in, energy burnt out. Simples! This diet and exercise regimen (as Vogue put it so eloquently: 'Exercise is a very important part of reducing'; what am I, gravy?) lasted precisely two days.

And so, of course, I never reached eight and a half stone. The magic number. The Holy Grail. The Goblet of Fire. The Half-Eaten Picnic. The moment my life will start, when I can turn a brand-new, pristine page unsplattered by tomato and mascarpone sauce, and I will finally, finally be happy. And be able to get a Topshop smock dress past my neck. Dear Lord, the other day I tried on a jazzy Clements Ribeiro horror in Evans, and, having been unable to get it on past my waist, I tried to get it off. Ooh, the pain. My ears are still bright red, and smarting.

8¹/₂ STONE

CHAPTER THREE
Transform your bathroom into a spa!

And so here I am, locked in the bijou avocado bathroom we've never been able to afford to update, on a weekday night. Bupi and Rav – the twins – are tucked up in bed: they share a room, as we live in south London, which despite the traffic congestion and the stabbings is now as expensive as Monaco, and had to graduate aged seven from bunk beds, as I was worried the top one would collapse (a house of cards or a garment factory in Bangladesh), and now have queen beds with a narrow gutter between them.

Most important fact to mention here is that it is my 30th birthday. You know that saying, you don't want to be fair, fat and 40? I figure if I get started on a new regime now and dye my hair I will be able to just about swerve that particular milestone. And so I am doing what all the glossy magazines tell me I should be doing and giving myself a 'spa night at home', indulging in some much-needed Self-Care on my Special Day, after what was frankly a disastrous date night with my husband, who is currently downstairs marking Year 4's homework.

I have lit candles everywhere. My phone is playing Native American plinky plonky music. I have floated rose petals I stole from next door's front garden in the water. I have unguents lined up, ready (and none of your cheap Garnier Fructose rubbish): a sugar/salt rub, a rose face mask, a pore strip for my nose that won't seem to adhere cos I'm sweating, foot and cuticle cream, a few fluffy warm towels and my sexiest nightie in the hope that tonight we finally have sex after a drought of, what, nine months? I could have made another human being in that time.

The steam, surely, is making the weight melt off me; I could be in Sweden, emerging in time for Newsnight resembling Agnetha from ABBA. I didn't have any dessert: the only bit of the birthday cake the twins bought me in M&S I actually ate was the icing stuck to the base of the candles (I'm afraid I made a rather unattractive sucking motion, a bit like Anthony Hopkins in The Silence of the Lambs; poor lambs). And so, for the first time in over a year, feeling crazily optimistic and giddy, I go to step on the scales. I swore I wouldn't weigh myself until I could fit into my skinny jeans – size 16, bought from Next to wear on my honeymoon; it was so bleeding hot, I couldn't get them up past my ankles.

It was exactly like that scene in Friends, where Ross uses lotion and talcum powder to pull on his leather trousers, only far, far more humiliating and messy – but, well, maybe the reason they still won't go past my calves is Neps put them on a hot wash along with his extreme fell running kit while I wasn't looking. Men are so annoying sometimes.

I take off my towelling dressing gown and my underwear; I swear, when I take off my bra it's like releasing two herds of cows to pasture. I step on the scales, breathing out; if coriander can cunting weigh something, I figure so can air. And I look. And I look again.

The needle is going crazy, whizzing from side to side in abject shock. Oh my God. No. Surely not. No. That cannot be right. I'm not pregnant with another set of twins, surely; they'd have come out by now. I kneel and fiddle with the dial, making damn sure the little bastard is bang on zero, remove each diamond stud from each ear, then try to remove my wedding band, without success: the cheap cunt doesn't need soap, it needs industrial cable cutters. Finally, in despair, I pinch each contact lens from my eyes, and flick. And peer again. Unfortunately, due to the steam and the sudden onset blindness, I can no longer see the tiny dial, and so I bend.

Not a good idea at the best of times. My body doesn't

really fold; it's like a very expensive mattress. Who knew the bathroom cabinet had such a hard edge? I can actually see stars. Perhaps I will have to buy a pair of scales that tells you your weight for next time: 'Pam. Seriously. You are morbidly obese. The likelihood of your husband fancying you, on a scale of 1 to 100, is minus 2. The probability of your foot being amputated due to diabetes is 2 to 1 odds-on favourite, but then at least you will weigh less.'

Finally, upset and near tears, bruised, nursing concussion, and just a teeny bit scared, I heave my bulk into the bath before it gets cold, displacing so much water the floor is now a swishing sea of petals and bubbles. This isn't self-care, it's self-harm. The moment spoiled, I heave myself out again, grab a bath sheet, and pat between the folds and truncated spurs and mountain ranges of my body – my stomach is a Viennetta, left too close to a two-bar electric fire – before giving in and putting on a winceyette nightie with a pie-crust collar. I resemble a lampshade.

I tiptoe downstairs, trying not to prompt Neps into thinking, 'Is it a T Rex or an Argentinosaurus huinculensis?' I am now in the sitting room. I cough. I put on another lamp. I pick up the remote and turn on Newsnight. I start hovering. I start hoovering. I spray the cushions with Febreze. And still he does not look up.

It must be the weight of those extravagant black

eyelashes that stops him acknowledging my existence. Are the essays of a 13-year-old inner city feral youth with attention deficit disorder and who has not yet been taught by his parents to use a knife and fork really that fascinating? On my Special Birthday Night? I wonder, not for the first time, if he really loves me. Because how can he love this. If I were a man, the sight of me naked would make me vomit. I want the best for him and I'm pretty sure that I'm not it. I wonder if he is ashamed of me. We have no mutual friends. We never invite people round for dinner; there never seems to be enough hours in the day or days in the week.

. . .

Actually, we did have a dinner party, once, when the twins were two. It was meant to be a celebration of his birthday, me having lost a bit of the baby fat, the twins at last sleeping through the night without needing me to raid the fridge for them. I'd raced home from work, done a supermarket sweep in the M&S on Brixton High Street and bought six bottles of wine. I had invited:

Izzy
Mum
The couple next door; I can't remember
their names

I kept asking Neps whom he was thinking of inviting.

Eventually, after much prodding and reminding and telling him 'I really need the numbers', which was like preparing for our wedding all over again, he reluctantly came back with:

Robert, a fellow teacher from school
His sister
His yoga teacher, a very bendy young man
named Niles, who later cancelled

I'd asked him at the time: 'Still no Rishi?' And he had shaken his head, mumbled something about him being caught up in his PhD. Rishi is his best friend from school. They met when they were eight. Rishi was always odd with me, even the first time he came to dinner at my house, when Neps and I first started dating. He'd taken his shoes off at the door, at my request, but as he descended to the kitchen his socks slipped and he crashed to the floor (he's not a small man). Turned out he broke a couple of ribs, was in agony for weeks. He didn't blame me, but Neps did: 'You and your OCD cleanliness when there's always cat hair on the dinner plates.' Rishi never came to the house again. But the oddest thing was when he refused Neps's invitation to be best man. I could only guess he couldn't stand the fact I was white. And unattractive. And overly house proud. And fat.

Mum couldn't come, as she was having a particularly

bad week, pain threshold-wise. Izzy bailed at the last minute – she really is a flake; mmm, Flakes. I really, really want one – as some man had asked her out to dinner instead. I said, well, bring him along, but she said all she really wanted to do was snort cocaine off his erect penis, which wouldn't really be welcome at the table as my twins might heave themselves down on their bottoms at 10 p.m. to beg for food. At half past seven I squished my way into the hallway, brandishing 18 M&S carrier bags. Neps was in the kitchen feeding the twins, who were confined in their high chairs.

'What have you got there?' he asked me, trying to sound enthusiastic but failing, massively.

'I went to Marks. Got a parsnip Wellington, lots of veggies to microwave, a tiramisu, lots of bubbly! Some cheese straws as canapés!'

'Um, ooh,' he said, hair bristling. 'Well, my sister doesn't drink. Neither does Niles. I have to be up early … And I was thinking of something more …'

'Indian? Made from scratch? Using a pestle and mortar? Should I have grown something from seed. Chillies, maybe? Garlic? Should I have converted our patio into a rice paddy? Built a greenhouse? Paid more attention during Gardeners' Question Time?'

'Well, yes.'

'I do have a job, you know.'

I probably say 'I do have a job, you know' 1,500

times a day, along with 'Neps? Neps? Neps?' I'm like a giant parrot. I sometimes think I should have a little recording saying those two things to save me the effort; I could just press a buzzer with my foot. And his bloody sister gets on my last nerve: she's a typical gap-year-taking millennial. The first time she came round after me and Neps got together – did I mention I'd already bought the terraced house? I got it cheap because it is in a slum clearance area and a prostitute was working from home next door – she had the cheek to say, 'Oh, hi. Are you, like, white, white?'

I'd asked her what exactly she meant.

'I mean, are you white, or is there something else in there that might, you know …'

'No, I don't know.'

'Well, like, if you were Italian, or French, or Spanish, that is not quite as bad as, like, white, white. We just read The Great Victorian Holocaust in Racism in History class at Nottingham Uni, so if you are white, white, i.e. English, you personally were responsible for a bigger Holocaust of my people, via Queen Victoria and Winston sodding Churchill, than what the Germans did to the Jews.'

I told her she should email Steven Spielberg, get him to make a blockbuster out of it with Liam Neeson as sort of a huge, pistol packing Mahatma Gandhi. I wish she weren't coming to this dinner. I really hope she has a heavy head cold or gets mugged by a huge black man on the walk here down the alleyway from the Tube.

'I have no idea why you wanted to do this,' Neps said, idly and ineffectually wiping the kitchen table. I noticed he was sweetly wearing the N.Peal cardi I'd given him that morning. I think he would get in the swing of things if only he'd drink alcohol; I really have no idea how people get through life without it. What else is there to look forward to at 6 p.m.? The twins were in their high chairs, long lashes casting shadows on their chubby cheeks, inky dhal leaking down their faces. They kicked their legs at the sight of me. I kissed them both – 'Ooh, that's spicy, Neps. Neps? Are you sure you didn't make it too hot for them, Neps? Neps?' – hoisting each one in turn out of their high chairs with the promise of a bath and a story and leftover tiramisu.

'Oh,' Neps said, unpacking bags with all the urgency of a sloth with a really bad hangover; I often wonder why I'm the only person in this relationship who has to do everything at top speed, in sixth gear with my foot down. 'Well, who is going to heat up this little lot? I've got some marking to do.'

. . .

And now, today, here we are on my momentous Special Night, and I am once again shouting 'Neps? Neps?!' Will someone please give me a little mirror, a tiny bell and a frond of millet?

Ooh, wait for it … Here come the eyelashes. As if in slow motion. Remember the Prince video for 'Alphabet Street'? No? Where have you been? Please YouTube it.

'Hmmm?'

I do not yet have his full attention. I do not have half his attention. I do not have a quarter of his attention. I have one segment of a Chocolate Orange of his attention. His eyes are still half-closed, lids enormous drawbridges belonging to some ancient King of the Far East who isn't quite sure yet whether he wants his quiet inner sanctum invaded.

'Neps?' I go to sit down. 'N—'

'Stop!' he shouts. Finally. I have the full beam of those huge dark eyes. 'You're about to sit on the cat!' I freeze, mid-lowering, and see the cat, tail a toilet brush, rocket out the room. Goodness. That was close.

I am sitting down now. Watching him. He really is beautiful: full lips, perfect white teeth without a single filling, inky black Kaia Gerber eyebrows, millimetre-long hair that always reminds me of iron filings. Oh, that I was a magnet.

'Yes? Are the twins in bed?'

'No. I've sent them to sew sequins on a frock for Primark. Of course they're in bleeding bed!'

He's changed out of the dark, narrow suit he'd worn to take me out to my disastrous birthday dinner and is in his off-duty uniform of oversize, low-slung sweats ('Which one are you?' I asked him once. 'Kriss or Kross?' 'How high do you want me to jump, jump?' he'd quipped back. You see, we did get on, once), tiny tight T-shirt and baseball cap that I swear he wears to hide his thoughts, not to mention jab me in the eye when I bend down to plant a dry peck goodnight.

'Look at you,' I say, plonking down on the other end of the sofa, which makes him lift a few millimetres into the air, for all the world as if we are at a playground instead of inside our two-up two-down shabby chic terrace with its sloping floors and rickety stair banister (the knob is always coming off in my hands) just off the mean streets of Railton Road. Out of habit, I pluck the nightie over my breasts (I have four breasts during the day, as even Curvy Kate's bras cut me horizontally in half, while at night I just have one big two-seater sofa with a corner bit that comes out when you pull a lever for your feet) and place a cushion on my tummy. I try to tuck my legs under me, and fail, so they loll, open, at my side. 'You look as though you've broken in to steal the telly, whereas I'm straight out of a Laura Ashley ad, circa 1982.'

'Did you enjoy your birthday dinner?' he asks me. To be honest, he had chosen a venue in the Barbican that most closely resembled a sandwich bar about to close.

'Um, yes, it was fine, once they took the tea towels and cling film off things.'

I choose not to mention the fact he had taken a book – A Suitable Boy: like me, it's really thick and solid and boring – with him and had actually got it out, surreptitiously, and placed it on his lap come the dessert course: a Skyr yogurt was the only thing on offer as Chef had, apparently, 'gone home'. When I asked him why he was reading he said that he was trying to take his mind off the sound of my chewing, as it was getting on his nerves.

'You haven't opened your presents,' he says, finally getting into the spirit of things now it's 11 p.m. He must feel sorry for me, as despite my best efforts my eyes are welling up and turning red.

He half gets out of his chair, reaches, and grabs two small packages and lobs them to me. Thank God for my two-ball skills. He is close, now, and I can see him gazing into my eyes. I almost break into Rod Stewart's 'Tonight's the Night'. But he stops. 'Have you been eating grapefruit again?'

'No, no. I got soap in my eye, that's all, during the spa at home thingy.'

I take the first gift and unwrap it. It is the aforementioned box of Harvey's Bristol Cream liqueurs. These dolly-sized bottles didn't even make my top 100, let alone the top 10! What is he thinking, anyway, giving me something I wouldn't give my mum, even if she didn't have diabetes on top of MS. But I can see he tried – he actually went inside a shop! And used his Electron card! And carried something towards the house! And found the Sellotape without asking me where it is first! – and so I unwrap a little bottle, and bite its head off, and sip, like Alice in fucking Wonderland. 'Trying to get me drunk?' I chortle. The sweet liquid runs down my chins.

'No, no,' he says, a little too quickly. 'I'm just trying to let you know that I don't spend every minute of every day worrying about your weight, the same as you do. There are other things in the universe to be concerned about. Perhaps you've found your natural level, so why fight it?'

This is a turn-up for the books. But I can't help but wonder silently why the change of heart. Does he really love me just as I am, or is he hoping I will keel over, like an oak tree after the storm of 1987, having ingested just one too many pyramid chickpea samosas in Masala Zone?

He snaps his laptop shut, puts the essays in a neat pile and back in his manbag, adjusts his baseball cap and yawns and stretches so extravagantly I see a sliver of dark-brown, hirsute tummy. I am impossibly, improbably aroused. 'I'm off to bed,' he says.

'But I've not opened the second gift yet,' I squeak. I know he paid for the twins' presents to me, unless they've been doing bob-a-job on the quiet: the cake, the onesie/duvet hybrid to put on for the brief nanoseconds when I'm not slaving away for minimum wage as PR for the biggest luxury brands in the universe.

'Oh, right,' he says, glancing extravagantly at his watch: Rolex, with a pale pink face, made in the year he was born, bought by me as his wedding gift. 'You know I have to be up for yoga in less than six hours.'

Jesus H. Christ. Yoga is Neps's secret weapon as a father of twins and husband of me. It is the ultimate get-out-of-jail card that can never, ever be trumped. Because he is Indian, from the Punjab, home of the Sikhs and hotbed of colonialism, I am not allowed because of political correctness and for fear of upsetting his ancestors and the Sikh god (he once, during an argument, asked me to name his ancestors; this, from a man who when asked to name my favourite designer said 'Next?' the cheeky cunt; he also had the cheek to say, when I tried on a new dress, that I 'look like Grayson Perry'), to ever, ever criticise the fact he devotes huge chunks of the day to the god of yoga. It is his birthright. It is not self-indulgent, girly exercise that costs loads and wastes time and creates washing when I barely have a moment to curl my eyelashes before assembling packed lunches and washing up breakfast while mopping the floor with the other hand while banking online and putting out the bins.

Because I am not allowed to be pastel pink, and princessy, and diva-ish, or ever, ever do a Beyoncé click of the fingers, and because I am so bloody lucky to have him as a husband given my size and racial profiling, I say, okay, I'll turn off the lights, don't you worry your little head. I still have a boil wash to put on, some trees in the road to pollard and the lawn to mow and the gutters to de-leaf.

I move slowly around the room, trying not to knock lamps off tables with my bulk, which precedes me by about four seconds. I put a couple of eggs on to hard boil for the twins' sandwiches. I have to scoop out the yolks and bind the white flesh with low-fat yogurt, because if child protection find any mayonnaise in the fridge alarms will go off and the twins will be seized and rehomed; at eight, they are not as big as I was at their age, but the Signs Are There: tummy crescents appearing from beneath T-shirts. The only difference from mine at their age is that their moon is light brown, cappuccino-coloured, not pearly white. One of the reasons I married Neps is I was hoping his DNA would trump mine, and I'm still not entirely sure it won't at some stage. Surely Bupi will start showing an interest in the three peaks soon, rather than buttering naans. Surely Rav will want to join the football team sometime soon, rather than wanting to stay indoors on Saturday morning 'in preparation for entering The Great British Bake Off'.

Back to the washing. I must load this blasted thing seven times a day. Sometimes, I think it's the only thing I do: in, out, in, out, shake it all about. I survey the small piles of clothes dotted around the kitchen floor. I plump for a dark wash – why not live a little for a change! – and start to feed the hungry machine, for all the world as though the navy gym knickers are mackerel and the machine a bored orca imprisoned in a joyless concrete tank. Secreted in the dark pile is a pair of Neps's jeans. Blimey. That's a first. They are not in a small concertina'd pile on the bedroom floor for once, left behind while he time travels. I hold them up, doing that motherly thing of going through pockets to retrieve coins and receipts and hankies. I never fail to wonder at the width of the hips, the sheer pencil-like quality. How can any human being fit in these? Where does it all go? What about his organs? His penis? And then I notice the hems are covered in mud, which has dried and is now spilling onto the floor. What on earth has he been doing? Ploughing? He, who is so fastidious he snaps the little clear lid onto his electric toothbrush head because he read somewhere the spray from the loo can travel up to six feet? I turn the jeans inside out, screw them up and bung them in, before pressing on the cycle that says 'Stains'. I stand, realising too late I have just stepped on the laundry capsule. It explodes everywhere. Damn. Honestly, it's as though I have three children.

And then I brace myself for the climb to bed. I actually lean on my knees on step two and then, anxious, jerk my head upwards in case he's looking down, watching my ascent, ready with winches and ropes and pickaxes and oxygen and criticism, like a Sherpa poised to heave the unfit white person in a helmet and Moncler jacket to the summit. But no. He's not there. Of course he's not. He's probably already asleep. Or reading on his iPad; sometimes I think the only reason he is glad when I get to bed is so he can use my back fat as a prop.

8$^1/_2$ STONE

CHAPTER FOUR
This doesn't work

I'm waiting for Izzy. Her office is in a mews house in Holland Park. The walls are lined with products made by the companies she represents. I never cease to be amazed at the ridiculous names: Drunk Elephant. Sunday Riley. (I must remember to complain to Mum, tell her she is too unimaginative and conventional. I'm sure if I were called North I wouldn't be outsize.) This Works, a brand dreamed up by the former beauty director of Vogue. As I scan the labels, each one promising to make me look less tired, ten years younger, to erase cellulite (I wonder if it would work on the cellulite on my arms?), to eradicate the seven signs of ageing (when I told Neps this was the reason I was spending up to 15 minutes every night basting my body with various creams at bedtime, he said, reasonably, 'What, loneliness, depression, arthritis, fuel poverty, dementia …?'). I wonder Izzy has the gall to peddle all this woo woo, to lie to beauty 'journalists', to bribe them with exotic stays in spas in Jamaica and Morocco, and then I begin to fantasise about launching a new brand myself, called 'This Doesn't Work'.

My gorgeous friend (she has the face of Halle Bailey, the body of Halle Berry; I, on the other hand, have the face of the Pillsbury Doughboy, the body of the Pillsbury Doughboy) is on speakerphone. (Why do people use speakerphone? Why not have a nice, quiet, normal conversation against your ear? When I asked Izzy this, she held her phone horizontally at arm's length and shouted, 'Radiation.' This from someone who smokes 20 full-strength Capstans a day.) Currently she also has a smoking acupuncture needle inserted in each lobe and is gazing at an iPad Pro, shouting to the agent's Executive Assistant No 3, 'Well, I'm sorry, but Tom Hardy is going to need a superyacht if you have a hope in hell of fitting on board his enormous PENIS.'

I'm used to overhearing these conversations, which all take place in a world where the Hotel Du Cap is the norm, rather than the local purple Premier Inn. While the world of PR I work in consists of me sending emails to bloggers along the lines of 'Dear ____, Are you doing any features on Christmas?', often forgetting to fill in the ____, Izzy is a portal to the stars, matching them with fabulous freebies (waterside seats for the Monaco Grand Prix, front-row gilt chairs for the Dolce & Gabbana cruise collection on the edge of Lake Como, access to the Vanity Fair post-Oscars party and the Serpentine Gallery Summer Party, Men's Finals day at Wimbledon), even though every one of her clients could afford to pay to attend all this stuff in designer gear without having to borrow it, and blag hotel stays, and Cartier earrings, and town cars. As always, the richer you are, the greedier you get and the less life costs you. Like most female PRs in our twenties, I have always supplemented my meagre wage by making sure I make the most of the fragrance launches, the backstage area at fashion shows, the inevitable after-parties: I would take five canapés at once, clamping my champagne flute in my armpit. I wonder if I should stop doing this; someone high up one day soon will find out I don't own a doggy for that bag. Last week, I was at a Versace after-party, queuing for the buffet, when a handsome man in a slim suit, a small microphone wrapped around his face as though he was about to join Madonna onstage, came up to me. 'Excuse me, Madame. Thees eez a private party. Are you an attendee, or are you …?'

I was so flummoxed by his quizzing that I lost my balance and some food tumbled to the floor. 'Oh no! I really wanted that risotto ball! What do you mean, of course I'm invited. I'm Miss, by the way, not Madame. And anyway, what makes you think I'm not a model?'

He had the cheek to smirk, before saying, 'About 20 stone … and about 20 years.' Cheeky bastard.

I realise I'm about to enter a downward spiral, doing what I always do: teetering off down memory lane to recall further slights and insults, line them up and relive them and feel upset anew.

Thankfully, finally, Izzy switches off her phone and turns the full beam of her fabulousness on me. I often think it's a good job her dark eyes are so huge, as there is simply so much of me to take in.

'Anyway, what do you mean you think Pi's having an affair?' (She always calls him this. I haven't even had time to see the film, let alone read the book.) She lets out a little growl and makes a swipe with an imaginary huge paw.

I'd told her, over a furtively typed text, that I think Neps might be cheating on me. There is no solid proof to speak of, no blonde hairs on his lapel, other than mine, no hotel receipts in his pocket (I looked, as you well know), but there have been Signs that only a wife would know.

First, m'lord and members of the jury, of course, is that we haven't had sex for nine months. I was organising a panel of male editors at a sort of male grooming festival, in between typing 'Dear ____', and in the lull while they had microphones pinned to Smedley fine gauge knitwear, I asked the editor of

Ps and Qs if it is normal for my husband and me not to have had sex for the equivalent of three quarterly bills from EDF.

'Hmm, well, he's having sex with someone,' he told me sagely and with a Roger Moore smirk. 'Just not with you.'

From the mouths of improbably happily, married-with-two-sons glossy fashion magazine editors who get their eyelashes permed …

Ever since then, I've been really worried. It's not just the lack of sex, or even the painfully slow lifting of the lashes: he's pretty much always done that. At our wedding breakfast, he didn't even sit next to me long enough at the 'top table' (bottom, more like) to make it past the starter before he was off, a lithe greyhound after a fake furry rabbit, to sling long arms round friends, to josh and to jape while I was left with a huge great gap next to me, a tramp's mouth after one too many Quality Street toffee pennies. (The worry has made me start eating again. It's all I can think about. It's all I live for.)

And then, as I explain to Izzy – not totally sure she is paying attention, as she keeps glancing at her Apple Watch and turning on her NutriBullet, and lighting another fag using the smouldering tip of the acupuncture needle (that's not allowed, surely? This must be the equivalent of going back on the

Hippocratic oath) – I was taking the twins to pick up Mum so we could all go to Meerkat World as Neps was away for the weekend on a geography field trip just outside Norwich, when a strange wrapper fell from the glove compartment. I'd picked it up, twisted to look at the twins strapped in the back. They were in matching tank tops, strained over tummies. Baby hands in laps. They haven't ever asked me for a phone or a tablet or even an Etch A Sketch or Fuzzy-Felt. They are like children from the fifties. They love the Famous Five, and pony books, and old Diana and Beano annuals snuffled out from Mum's wardrobe. Which is all fine, except for the fact she can't help but overfeed them. Even at Meerkat World, having agreed they could have a lolly, she had yelled up at the ice cream man in his van, 'Can they have two scoops, and a Flake, and a cone?' Finding the wrapper, I'd asked the twins if their gran had been secretly feeding them meat behind my back. 'No, Mummy!' they'd piped in unison. 'But she does sometimes order a McDelivery when you're late home from work.'

Anyway, upon mention of finding something untoward in my outwardly cosy marriage, I find I have her attention, and she looks up from her wrist. 'What? A condom wrapper? He's having sex with other women in your car! But it's a hatchback!'

'No. Not a condom. A pork pie wrapper. A really

cheap brand, as well.'

Now, Izzy is a committed Plant Eater, and so doesn't eat meat or even dairy, 'unless blow jobs count'. And Neps is a Sikh, which means he too is vegetarian. I have converted (not to Sikhism, but to not eating animals – except on Christmas Day, when if I didn't eat the turkey cooked and untiringly basted by Mum for the last 14 days she would threaten to wheel her chair into the Serpentine), thinking being vegetarian might help me lose weight, and the twins of course have been brought up veggie. Which can only mean one thing. He has had a woman in the car who grew ravenous after sex. He would never, ever let me eat meat in the car, or anywhere else.

'Could it be a colleague?' Izzy asks me reasonably. 'A friend? You can't really accuse him of cheating on you because of one measly pork pie wrapper. What is this, a game of Cluedo? Who d'ya think done it? Colonel Mustard? Miss Scarlet Woman?'

'It's not just that. He is very distant. It's as though I'm an annoyance he puts up with. Even when we had Birthday Sex—'

'Ah. So it hasn't really been nine months …'

'No, but the main point of being married, apart from children and someone to help pay the mortgage, and go up ladders, and rescue insects from the bath, and turn out dozy bumblebees, is that you are guaranteed he will have to have sex with you on your birthday and kiss you at midnight on New Year's Eve: a proper kiss, not a dry, testudinal peck. That's the deal. It's compulsory. It's written into the vows. Anyway, even during Birthday Sex he had his eyes closed. He didn't realise he was smothering me with my own breasts.'

'Oh dear.' Izzy looks puzzled. She too has large breasts, but they are entirely man-made and so defy all the rules of physics. 'Then what happened?'

'Well, I almost passed out. I was re-enacting that bit with Elizabeth whatsit in The Abyss: officially dead and having to be reinstated by Ed Harris.'

She laughs, then swoons. 'Oh God, I'd love to have mouth-to-mouth from Ed Harris, have him pound on my chest.'

'And then he sloped off to the bathroom, presumably to have a big old wank. The other day, he said without make-up I look like someone with Down's Syndrome. He tried to pass it off as a joke, but still ... I think the bag is putting him off.'

'What, did you treat yourself how I told you to in Selfridges the other day? You know you're worth it.'

'No. The Bag.' I realise my mouth is making a Dick Emery curl. I can't help it. 'Down there.'

She is fascinated. 'Let me look!'

And so, against my better judgement, I show her. The white flap of skin a pitta bread that has forgotten to be griddled. Soft and floppy and dimpled, hanging over my bright-pink M&S pants.

'Oh my God,' she says, and goes to lift it, as though it were some sort of dead sea animal, then thinks better of it, recoils, shudders. 'How on earth does he ever find … you know?'

'Well, he has lifted it in the past, and it is almost as though he's a postman, afraid of a drooling, aggressive German Shepherd on the other side.'

She honks with laughter.

'It's not funny.'

'Does he still, you know, go down …'

'Oh no. He doesn't. Not anymore. I find it boring, on the whole, but here's another thing.' I gather myself on her Wassily chair to my full height and clasp my arms beneath my bosoms, for all the world as though we are pegging out washing in the ginnel wearing aprons and curlers. 'Before he submerged me under 72 metres of my own flesh, he did have a go, down there [Dick Emery, again; I really wish he would go away], because it was my birthday, and he had a whole new technique. Someone had obviously taught him how to do it. I almost came.'

'He could have Googled it.'

'No. A woman just knows. A wife has a sixth sense. Radar. We're like dolphins. Or bats.'

Izzy raises both microbladed brows. She has never been married, and I doubt she ever will. Much to her

African parents' chagrin, she has always favoured posh white boys, while I, as we know, have gone the other way. What is the name of that box of chocolates that is half milk, half plain? Why, even in times of crisis, do I think of everything in terms of cocoa solids?

She chooses to ignore my marital status and says instead, 'When I asked my last boyfriend to spank me, he screwed up his face and whined that his mum didn't camp for a decade at Greenham Common and grow her armpit hair just so her son could oppress women; he offered to refuse to pay the bill at dinner! Fucking feminists have ruined it for the rest of us!'

I wonder, not for the first time, if Izzy is so into sex, with so many men, as a way of getting back at her strait-laced parents. She used to take a lot of cocaine, too. I remember she got very involved with a man in New York, David, who was seriously into coke. 'He's great in bed, set to inherit a fortune; permanently dripping nose, but apart from that really handsome!' was how she described him. I can't understand how she is still single, given she's so beautiful and well connected. In one of my more depressed moments, I tell her I think she might have been a better match for Neps, at which she honks with laughter. 'Listen, he's a little Punjabi boy who struck gold with you. If he was married to me, I'd have to move in with him and his parents, sit on the floor and make chapattis and children. Eurgh.'

She once got me a personal trainer as a birthday gift. He used to turn up at my house in Brixton, looking nervous, to take me on a power jog. In those days, if you went running in Brockwell Park it was because a youth in a hoodie with a knife was after you. In the end, I tipped a bowl of washing-up water over his head.

I appreciate her efforts, I really do. But I am still the size and shape of a bungalow – with a conservatory – so nothing has worked.

'I know Neps has gone off me because I'm fat ...'

'Not morbidly so ...'

'What planet are you on? When I was on the bus yesterday, people thought I was mit Baby!'

'I'm not that interested in children,' she says, smartly bringing the conversation back to being All About Her. 'I just don't think they're a good idea,' she adds, probably forgetting, again, that I have two rather large kiddies stashed at home. 'Look what happened to Sadie Frost! Plus, how could you guarantee they would turn out attractive, despite the gene pool? Look at the Beckham brood! They make my eyes hurt. Plus, look at what childbirth does to your body! Miley Cyrus, "Wrecking Ball" anybody?'

She looks me up and down as she says this last bit. I think about being offended, but then I give in. I'm here for honesty and pragmatic woman-on-woman advice, not for her to shore me up with all those lies girls tell each other to avoid you hacking at your wrists with a pink Lady Shave, advice which never, ever bloody well works anyway:

'A mullet is perfect on a wedding dress.'

'He is going to ring you, please don't worry, he's probably just busy, or abroad, or dead.'

'Perhaps he's saving up to buy you something better, and this one is just a token? Your finger isn't that green, anyway. You wouldn't notice, unless you're looking for it.'

'His mum does like you, she's just old and senile and probably suffers from Tourette's.'

'I'm sure he ends all his work emails with several xxxx's and a smattering of red hearts, accompanied by a virtual explosion of rose petals and fireworks.'

'Of course he enjoyed sleeping with you. Maybe he always says to women "Thank you for your support."'

'Perhaps he's just shy.'

'I'm sure he's thinking of marriage. Just because he says, "You take care" when he leaves your dinner date at 8.10 p.m. doesn't mean he's giving you the brush-off. He could have a really hungry cat.'

'Alexander Wang always comes up a bit small. It's not you. It's him.'

'He wasn't ignoring you; he just forgot his glasses and the restaurant was really foggy from people vaping.'

'I know my body is ravished, ravaged, ruined,' I tell her. 'I let myself go after the twins were born; well, during pregnancy, really, and before conception, if truth be told. I always thought I might resemble Demi Moore, naked on the cover of Vanity Fair, then realised they'd probably need a gatefold.' She's heard me say this before, so I add to get her attention, 'I can never tell when he's inside me, not now I've had twins. I imagine he stopped wanting sex because he got fed up with the constant wailing, "Is it in, or is it out?" He was starting to feel like a bleeding tennis umpire at Wimbledon. "Shall I go and fetch a really high stool?" he said once, before going off in a mood.' She honks again.

'Plus, my career is going down the pissing pan, probably because I'm so worried about Neps I've taken my eye off the ball. I must be the only woman in the world who has managed to sleep her way to the bottom. We had our morning blue-sky meeting the other day and all my boss could think about was why I wear so much stretchy black – "Has somebody died?" she asked me; yeah, only my ambition – and what would Philip Green think if he could see me, and how I'd turned from a pear into a watermelon or a pumpkin, that sort of thing. She says she's thinking of moving my desk inside the stationery cupboard, as when clients come in for a meeting and see me, growing there, I am apparently "blurring the brand message". She's already banned everyone from eating at our desks; who does she think she is, Anna bleeding Wintour?'

'Well, that's bullying. You should MeToo her.'

'I'm to come up with a strategy for rebranding Philip at London Fashion Week, post his plummeting profits that no one is allowed to talk about in case he rescinds our 40% discount cards, but I don't think I have the strength to stand outside Somerset House in the rain, wielding an iPad, while 12-year-olds who blog step over my huge dead body.'

'At least if you're dead you'll be a skeleton,' she says sensibly. Adding a rather cruel and Spanish accented, 'H'e-van-tu-ally.'

I tell her that I plan to be cremated, thank you very much: I want to increase global warming to get my revenge on the injustices of the world. Plus, that I am definitely going to join the gym. Tomorrow. She looks aghast: 'Gyms are like NHS hospitals: teeming with superbugs. Have you ever seen a guy use a wet wipe after he has finished secreting over everything?'

'No, I know, never. It's laziness. They go to the gym to avoid emptying the dishwasher and eye contact.'

Izzy has always really tried to help me lose weight (which is more than I can say for the girls in the office, sample size to an idiot). She once gifted me Roxanne, a woman in Venice Beach who was a 'wisdom holder', whom Izzy guaranteed 'would help me deepen into myself via guided contemplations'. Roxanne, after making me answer millions of questions on an online form, curated me a self-help reading list via email and sent me a shopping list so I could subsist off home-made smoothies: chia seeds, agave nectar, unwaxed lemon juice. She sent me a Daily Menu and Ground Rules ('commit to one hour a day of transformative daily mind practice, pick a book about transformative thinking, go on a negativity diet' – now, that's one diet I haven't yet tried!) and told me to 'ask the universe a question'. Okay, here we go, answer this one, oh dear unending, unfathomable, unknowable galaxy (ooh, Galaxy Counters): 'Why the fuck in God's name am I fat?' She also sent me an Intention Contract, Shopping List, Salt Water Flush, Veggie Power Juice Recipes (the Hardcore Green Juice was actually quite nice, akin to inhaling a hedgerow in summer), Coffee Alternatives and, finally, Raw Soup Recipes, as well as a packet of detox stuff to sprinkle on my bathwater. She used to email me every morning, saying things like, 'Add a little pizzazz to your water with cucumber slices, a sprig of rosemary or unwaxed lime juice!' I ended up wanting to stab her overly positive visage with a rusty serrated knife.

Roxanne's most oft-repeated nugget of advice was for me to 'complete one difficult task a day'. I do 500 difficult things before 9 a.m.! While juggling and standing on one leg! One difficult task?! One?! What planet is she living on? She obviously doesn't have children, and works from home, and is dating a man who when asked to put up a picture on the wall doesn't respond with, 'Can it not just sit on the floor?'

Izzy starts to fidget and pull on her coat, and order an Uber, and turn off lights, and set the alarm, which is generally a sign I've outstayed my welcome.

'Got any freebies I can have?' I ask her, putting my phone, which hasn't vibrated once all day, the passive aggressive little shit, back in my bag. Neps used to leave little poems in my suitcase when I went away on press trips; my favourite, which I kept and had framed (it's still sitting on the floor), read: 'I know I'm grumpy but please don't dump me, I have to have you so why not hump me?'

These days, the only notes from him are the ones he Post-its on the fridge: 'Can no one touch my green smoothie? Thanks.' It's as though we're flatmates. If we were friends at school, I'd have gone from getting a Christmas card with glitter and a 3D kitten in snow, to something monochrome featuring Mary and Jesus. The other day, snooping on his Facebook page, I noticed his relationship status says: 'It's complicated'.

I'm still molesting her products while she's preparing to exit her office with a checklist that would rival that of an astronaut destined for Mars. 'C'mon, Izz. Stuff for stretch marks. Or a phial of serum for someone who's been badly burnt in a wildfire and lost their home?

Or for after a long stretch of chemo? I'm feeling really stressed. I think my telomeres have started fraying.'

I remove a cheese and onion pasty from my bag, almost without realising I'm doing so, and start to chomp. 'Ew,' I say, remembering the pasty is really old, examining it for green signs of mould before taking another huge bite and chewing miserably.

'Honestly, you are the limit,' she says, taking it from me and lobbing it out the window. I go to object but realise she's right. The other day, in Carluccio's (seriously, it's a sea of nannies as beautiful and wholesome as Kate Upton; I got caught up in all the prams and buggies by the door; I was a whale shark, snared in a net, drowning), she coughed, and a bit of her breadstick landed on the table between us and I reached over and *put it in my mouth*. Then she says: 'Did you ever wear the reiki sweater, by the way, y'know, the cashmere one impregnated with good vibes? I gifted it to you last season.'

'Um …'

'Did you keep it in the gold pouch between wears to keep the healing intact like I told you? Did it not work? Maybe this is why all this bad stuff is happening to you. Oh, and did I tell you that, Stella McC-fashion, you must not wash it, as that would leach away the positive energy …'

'Er, no, sorry, I didn't wear it. The label said XXL

but I couldn't get it past my neck.'

'Shame. I always have an interesting night out when I'm wearing mine, though when I wear the red version people do tend to get confrontational around me ...'

Suddenly, she puts everything down, removes the acupuncture needles from each lobe, and blows on them – Puff! Puff! – for all the world as though she is Mae West starring in a cowboy movie.

'I've got it!' she says, Rex Harrison-fashion. 'I am going to make you over. You are going to be my renovation project. I am going to be Alan Titchmarsh, faced with a mountain of solidified concrete and a disabled person! I am going to gift you Mr Kalimares!'

CHAPTER FIVE
Don't you dare Instagram this!

Which is why, precisely two weeks later, I'm at the St John and Elizabeth private hospital in leafy and very posh St John's Wood, wearing my best navy knickers and nothing else bar a few great big sweeps of a frankly cold and petrol smelling felt-tip pen.

An Egyptian surgeon is still wielding the felt-tip pen, as though he is an overgrown toddler in a messy activity class, pondering his handiwork and deciding which colour to choose next from its Caran d'Ache pouch. It's weird, isn't it, how someone whose prime objective is to get through the day without anyone seeing a centimetre of bare skin, who pulls cardis over breasts, and sweaters down over the shelf that is my bottom, and pashminas around upper arms, and scarves up over chins, and plonks cushions on tummies, can very quickly adapt to being near-naked, given the right set of circumstances? Your first extreme bikini wax, for example. Hello, how are you? Are you busy today? Hold both knees up and splay; of course, no problem. Do you want the inner lips done? Yes please! Can you place one hand on each buttock and pull them apart? Absolutely! Planning any holidays this year?

Childbirth. I think childbirth is a slippery slope. I should never have told Neps which hospital I was delivering them in; I'm reminded of that fabulous Bridget Jones line: for a man, witnessing his wife give birth is like finding out his favourite pub has burnt down. I should have said I was popping out for some logs or something, not squeezing two humans – two overcooked humans, if truth be told (two-and-a-half weeks late! I'm going to apply for compensation) – from between thighs which, as you can probably imagine, have no gap at the top. My legs are so fat at the top, people have mistaken me for a mermaid or – and this is a more common response – a giant slug. We should have just bought two tiny infants from Neps's parents' village in the Punjab, not made them from scratch. We buy cauliflower, after all. Potatoes. We don't have to grow them.

So, I blame the twins, really, for why I'm here in this pristine white room, with Izzy brought along as backup, Starsky to my Hutch, only with better knitwear. She is watching proceedings with great interest and an iPad at the ready. 'Don't you dare Instagram this!' I spit at her as she goes to raise her screen just at the precise moment the surgeon lifts up my breasts, just to make sure I'm not hiding any sandwiches under there. Izzy is a huge fan of plastic surgery, having had her ample breasts lifted and her nipples made smaller, so they now resemble two teeny pink flying saucers (the sweet made from rice paper, not the ones made by aliens). I only realise when Mr Kalimares replies that I said the thing about blaming my children out loud.

'Now, Mrs Dhariwali. You do realise that if you are going to have a tummy tuck, that it is best you do so after you have finished making your family? It is a dangerous, expensive, painful procedure. It is best not to even contemplate having another baby after I have reattached your abdominal muscles.'

What planet is this man on?

'My husband no longer fancies me, so it is highly unlikely I am ever going to have sex again. Let alone get pregnant.'

I start to sweat, and he asks if I'm nervous, having second thoughts. 'No, just cut the bag off!' I get hot everywhere. It's one of the drawbacks of being overweight. People assume I'm menopausal. I really didn't need the prospect of global warming coming along and worrying me.

He tells me I have to understand why I gained weight so I don't pile it all back on after surgery. I consider saying that we still don't know why there are black holes, or how the universe started, and that the reason some people get fat and others don't is third on the unknowable list when Izzy interrupts.

'Tell him about your polycystic ovaries. Go on. Victoria Beckham has them, too: bad skin, thin hair, moody, tendency to gain weight …'

'I know all about Victoria Beckham, thanks very much. And I don't have thin hair. That's all very well, but how about the poly-Twixes my mum force-fed me to compensate for the fact my dad left us? I know all this. I know why I could never lose weight as a child, why it was so hard to conceive the twins. I'm a bleeding world expert! It doesn't change the fact—'

The surgeon interrupts me in full flow. I'm quite impressed, actually, by how disinterested he is in the logistics or the emotions. To him, I am simply a fillet of steak, just waiting for him to excise the gristle with his chef's knife and smack me on the griddle with some chanterelles.

'Your stomach muscles have divided, Red Sea-fashion, to make room for the stress-fat mummy tummy. I will have to sew them back together. Here, and here.

'Once I have knitted the muscles together, I then excise the flap of skin, which will never disappear without surgery, even with exercise – even if you qualify for the pommel horse at the Olympics, ha ha ha! – and sew you up. While you are still under general anaesthetic – why not? Ay ay, seize the moment! – I will perform liposuction here, here and here; and here and here and over there and under that bit, that bit, ooh, nearly missed that bit, oh dear, that one's nasty! Once a fat cell has formed it will always be there and so sucking them out is the only way to get rid of them. Dieting just shrinks them; they lurk, waiting to puff up the moment you even sniff a tiramisu. But I must warn you, liposuction is not a simple solution: it's painful, there's bruising, and swelling …'

I tell him I don't care. That I cannot live like this a moment longer. With the huffing and the puffing, the folds, the moist seams, the cress, the stress, the looks I get if ever I dare set foot inside a shop, any shop, even Boots. My big fat body is all anyone ever sees. All I want to do at the moment is get through the day until I can trundle upstairs to bed. Under the covers, just my eyes peeking over the top of the duvet, is the only time I feel normal and safe.

And then the surgeon does something amazing and miraculous. He frogmarches me to the full-length mirror, an oblong object I've been shunning since I spotted it when we first came in. (I've always hated mirrors: at high school, I would slide towards the basins along a wall in the girls' loos and never look up; this is part of the reason I hate hotels: so many unfriendly mirrors that jump out at you like muggers or rapists, mirrors you've not yet learned how to avoid or befriend or pout past.) Then carefully and gingerly he lifts the pitta bread bag to show me what the effect will be post-op.

And there – oh my God! – is the navy triangle of my knickers. I haven't seen that properly since I was 21! And oh, as I twist to see it from different angles, it all looks so much better, more normal: I am still Jabba the Hutt, but no strange bag of skin, a yawning empty room like the one when the twins finally go off to uni, please Jesus and thank the Lord, while this nice, gentle, capable, highly trained man holds the flap up.

'I might just ask you to follow me around forever!' I say, almost twirling. 'It would be like valet parking. My own personal flap holder!'

He unhands me at last. I feel deflated, suddenly very down indeed. The flap is back, boom, like an impenetrable portcullis. I don't want to sound ungrateful, but I have to know whether I will have a scar where the bag has been cut off. I still haven't told Neps that I am getting a tummy tuck, as I'm not sure how he will react. Will he worry about me going under a general anaesthetic, or will he be angry he'll be left in charge of the twins and the hard egg boiling? Will he be able to tell I've had something done, or will he just believe that my one, solitary visit to the gym last year (to buy a sandwich) reaped results?

'You will have a scar, my dear Pam, but it will fade in time. You will have to wear a corset for three months, to support the muscles. [Oh God no, he'll notice that! On second thoughts, though, he didn't notice the other night that I had a huge bruise on my head from all the birthday weighing while blind. I sometimes wonder if he'd recognise me in a police line-up. 'Mr Dhariwali. Can you point out the figure of your wife?' 'Um … Er …'] Don't worry, the nurse will tell you what to expect and what to do. We will give you a special oil for the scar, but it will be hidden beneath the line of your bikini bottom, so …'

I almost faint with shock. I hug him, rather clumsily imprinting some red felt tip on his immaculate white coat. 'I will be able to wear a … bikini??!!!!!!'

. . .

All this talking about two-pieces reminds me of my honeymoon. I think I had PTSD. I know I'm still paying off the credit card bill.

I was stressed to begin with, even when we landed at the airport. (Although isn't it lovely when they open the plane door, and you step onto the metal stairs and sniff, and it feels completely different: hot and moist and fragrant and full of possibilities?) I was so worried about whether my cheque for the buffet at the Trinity Square pub would bounce, I kept scrolling my texts for any that said, 'Low balance alert' and 'Please come to debtors' jail'. Neps, of course, on his left-wing teacher's wage (he is always really rude about my career, putting on an insipid voice when I say I'm tired and could he put the Linda McCartney in the oven, saying, 'Are you planning any features for Valentine's Day?'), only contributed the cost of his very nice, very narrow-cut Dior Homme suit by Hedi Slimane (slim by name, slim by nature), shirt, tie and socks by Timothy Everest and shoes by Churchill.

The wedding was worth it, though. Neps's aunties persuaded Mum to wear a bright sari, despite her consternation that it would reveal a generous slice of tummy; for once, though, we weren't the fattest women in the room. All his aunties and cousins had spare tyres, and they were all completely unashamed of exposing them. Perhaps what's wrong isn't me, it's just that I live on the wrong subcontinent. His uncles pushed Mum from Brixton Town Hall to the pub in her wheelchair at great speed; all I could hear as I de-podded myself from the taxi was her squealing with joy, pink and lime fabric streaming behind her, shouting, 'It's like The Far Pavilions!' Come midnight, we were all dancing to Bollywood tunes in the room above the bar.

The long-haul flight was a mistake, as we were both still tired, but I had got a good deal on an all-inclusive holiday in Mauritius. On landing, though, my panic and sense of foreboding was compounded by the fact that when we went to pick up the hire car it turned out Neps had passed his test too recently – he cycles everywhere, in Spanx; but you already knew this – to be able to drive it. Which meant I was the one who had to squeeze behind the steering wheel of a car obviously built for tiny Mauritian people the size of elves and drive on the wrong side of the road while the wedding bubbly was still secreting from my pores.

I was also worried the pre-wedding grooming regime – waxing (half leg, underarm, under other arm, Extreme Bikini), gel pedi and mani, facial threading including nostrils (v painful), lash and brow tinting, facial, micro dermo-whatsit and the non-taking on board of water – was starting to wane and I was beginning to go off. By day two, it was like that moment in a horror film where the sky goes pink and you happen to be a vampire and you've lost your door key. I was worried the bright, tropical sunlight was highlighting everything I didn't want to be highlighted with great big Hollywood searchlights: stray chin hairs, orange-peel skin, badger stripe of regrowth on head, bank balance, my tonsils. I wonder if my tonsils are fat or if they're normal.

Neps, on the other hand, took to tropical island life like a very swimmy duck to a pond. Baggy, Rafa Nadal shorts pulled on in a jiffy, bare, hairless pecs, iron-filings hair glistening from the outdoor shower, exotic birds fluttering around him as though he were a human in a Disney cartoon. And you know that trick men have to find someone, anyone, to champion over you, wherever they go – taxi driver, waitress, postman, bin man, road sweeper, DHL delivery man, even the old woman in a headscarf at traffic lights who tries to clean your windscreen? – Neps soon, by our first morning as a married couple (does 'S'pose we'd better consummate it' and rubbing his hands together count as talking dirty?), discovered he was best and undying and lifelong mates with the resort staff, with whom he decided to play football, and rain with gratuities, and give away his box-fresh trainers to, BOUGHT BY ME FOR THE HONEYMOON. They, of course, were the proletariat, the deserving, the underdogs, the righteous, while I, having gone to an all-girl grammar and once played netball, was the Oppressor. The Bitch. The Colonialist.

All of which meant I ended up having breakfast, every day, on my own. Other holidaymakers would approach my table and I would think, 'Oooh, a new friend to talk to,' and lift my head and smile expectantly and warmly, only for them to make off with any spare chairs. But it wasn't all bad, as it was an All-You-Can-Eat-Without-Exploding buffet, and Neps's new-found passion for barefoot soccer and volleyball meant there were no Disapproving Eyes as I piled on more granola (healthy, no?) and pineapple carpaccio. The only sad bit was when I spied a humming bird and had no one to um and aah and point it out to.

By day two, it all started to go Very Wrong Indeed. Despite spraying on Sisley Sun Barrier factor 75, I started to go bright pink, like a flamingo, only not quite as etiolated. The heat brought me out in hives, which being nearer the sun also became very red, while my ankles puffed up like bouncy castles. My sarong – or, as Izzy called it, my 'pareo', having couriered it to me at Heathrow when I'd told her I'd forgotten to bring a wrap, but instead had bought a pair of grey linen drawstring trousers from Per Una ('Do you want Chinese people to hunt you down and lop bits off you to grind down into a powder?') – had started to stick to my body in a shroud. It was the afternoon and I was sat at a small table on the beach, trying to see if I could make out the form of my new husband using the concierge's whale-spotting binoculars, when he hove into view, dribbling a football.

As he approached my table, I immediately sat up straight and sucked in my stomach, trying to smile and not look too needy or purple while hiding my ice cream behind a cactus. I twirled my wedding band and the engagement ring. I was so proud. I was one of those annoying women with diamonds on their ring finger. I was no longer a pariah. The unloved. Single. Someone adored me enough to put a ring on it, even if it was £79.99 from H Samuel, the stone so small it could be classified as a 'chip' (oh God, chips). Who wants to be one of those ladies who lunch (oh God, lunch; when is it?) with engagement rings the size of hippos married to bankers they never see. They are no better than common prostitutes.

He waved, for all the world as though I were his dear old mother, beached on the shore buttering rolls and diluting Kia-Ora, and then, just as I thought he was about to dribble away and I could at last breathe out, the ball shot under my table, getting stuck. He took an age to fetch it, using only his feet, the annoying arse, then cantered away, ball tucked under his sinewy, twiglety arm, and gave me a backwards glance just in time to see me breathe out, stomach sending champagne glass, table, parasol, telescope, ice cream and pareo flying.

He returned slightly towards me, shaking droplets photogenically from his head as though he were an otter emerging from a river. I thought he was coming to help me clear up. 'You need to be careful of all that broken glass,' he said. 'Most of the staff here can't afford shoes.'

I'm still not sure whether to go through with it. I have had my pre-op appointment and consultation, where the nurse, a beautiful young Iranian lady called Jasmine, took little phials of blood (I kept telling her to take more, to make me weigh less; 'Here, have an armful!') and listened to my heart, took my blood pressure and all that sort of thing. Even with a press discount arranged by Izzy, I am looking five grand in the face. I have no idea where I am going to get five grand from; I will have to get a loan. I've been looking at my direct debits, wondering which ones I can cancel: gym membership? Yes. Sky TV? Yes. The Times subscription. Yes. Life insurance. Hmmm. I look up the policy. Blimey. I am worth more dead than alive.

Plus, of course, I am going to have to take 2 weeks off work. The only person I decide to tell, other than Izzy, is Mum. So, after work on a Monday, which is the only evening Neps doesn't have some sort of physical activity lined up, I drive along the busy A127 to see her. She has made me a cup of milky tea and has placed a chocolate biccie on the saucer. No, Arthur Lee of sixties psychedelic band Love. You are very, very wrong. Forever never bloody well changes.

She isn't happy when I gently but firmly break the news of my impending tummy tuck and bag removal and liposuction. She's worried about the expense, how

Neps will cope, what the twins will think and, lastly and most importantly, about the dangers of any such invasive surgery: 'You could catch MDMA.' But Mrs Malaprop more than anyone knows what I've been through, because she went through it first. It's funny, isn't it, how much we take after our mums, without even realising: I only buy green Fairy Liquid, never yellow or red. I bank with NatWest. I put a washed cheese grater under the grill to make sure it's dry. I put clothes pegs on the top of open packets of food. I put my floor mop in the garden to air. And I have a BMI of 297.

I haven't, though, uttered a word to alert her to my doubts about Neps: worry makes her condition much, much worse, and I have already offloaded enough. Plus, I am slightly dreading an element of 'I told you so'. If I mention my theories that he's cheating it would turn into the inevitable wailing and thrashing. But being Mum, she has a sixth sense about these things. 'You're not doing this for Him, are you? I always told you that you and whatshisname [she has never, ever got his name right, and doesn't even go there with our surname, Dhariwali] were too different. It's not being racist to say that he's from a different culture, so he's never going to understand ours. Or you.'

'Mum, we don't have any culture.'

'Yes, we do. Morecambe and Wise. The pier. His dad ate the main with his fingers at the wedding do.' (We'd had Indian-themed canapés and a sitar player, who was sadly drowned out by all the chatting; I almost asked for my money back.)

'Mum. His dad's a dentist. His mum has a PhD. Neps could have done a master's if he hadn't got manacled to me.'

'He is very lucky to have you,' she says. 'And those gorgeous children, whatever their names are.'

'I know there are risks in surgery, Mum, but it's dangerous being this big, too.' I pick up my cup and ostentatiously remove the biccie as though it were a stray cat hair, but I can't help but lick the chocolate that has melted on the side. Old habits die, ooh ... maybe I should become a nun. They don't care what they look like, they wear long scratchy outfits, they are married to a dead man. Maybe that's the way to go; cheaper, too. I continue: 'Neps doesn't fancy me anymore and who can blame him? I'm like the mother in What's Eating Gilbert Grape? I know what's eating Gilbert Grape: it's me.'

'You're too self-depreciating,' she says, her eyes moist. 'You are lovely. Kind. Thoughtful. Bubbly.'

She starts to cry, which I can't bear. I try to hug her and get about halfway: round about South Africa.

'But we know more now,' she says, sniffing ostentatiously. 'You don't give the twins sweets ...'

'I think it's in their genes, written in their DNA.

And I know they're ashamed of me. I don't want them to have a fat mum. Look at what happened last sports day? I couldn't fit inside the sack. I came last in the egg and spoon.'

She gives me an old-fashioned look. 'Yes, but that's because you kept stopping to peel the egg and nibble it.'

. . .

Driving back to London, I am beginning to have second thoughts. Mum was so worried – the cost, the dangers, the motives – that I feel I need to talk it through with someone … not exactly neutral, but obviously someone who is completely on my side.

And so, while I'm at a traffic light, I dial Izzy.

'Izz. Can you meet me this evening? I've just told Mum my surgery plans and she's not happy. I need to talk it through with someone.'

'Have you told Neps yet?'

'No. That's another thing. I'm not sure how to do it. He is bound to moan about wasting so much money and him having to look after the twins and learn how to change the Hoover bag.'

'Okay, listen, can you meet me at the Sanderson?'

I tell her that is perfect and I jab the postcode into my phone. I can't go home, not yet. I need to make a decision.

I manage to park just off Oxford Street and make my

way to the hotel. It is stuffed full of white, diaphanous net curtains and white, diaphanous people. I go up to the bar, displacing glamorous couples with my bulk. I feel as cumbersome as a snowplough; someone should accessorise me with orange flashing lights. I spy Izzy in the garden, smoking. She waves, stamps out her ciggie and comes in.

'What are you drinking?' she asks me.

'Oh no, nothing. I'm driving, plus I need a clear head.'

She orders champagne for her and a virgin cocktail for me. Plus some nuts. 'Last meal,' she says, shoving the tiny bowl towards me.

I tell her how worried Mum is, how I am having second thoughts.

'Listen,' she says. 'This is a first for you. But Mr Kalimares performs this procedure every single day. It is normal for him. Completely routine.'

'Yeah, I guess. It's just that I'm scared.'

She orders another drink. The place is so loud I can barely hear myself think. I check my phone. No text from Neps asking where I am. I might as well be dead. And as I sit there, watching young women with shiny hair in minidresses snaking past, smiling, flirting, laughing, I decide: I want to be like them. I want to be happy. I am going to go through with it.

'Good for you,' Izz says. 'And I have a date!'

'But it's 10 p.m.!'

'I know! Early! It's all the way over in Reading, FFS ...'

'Ah, the hedge fund bloke and his mansion.'

'Yeah. There will be a few people there, but I'm hoping.'

She stands, unsteady in her heels. She must have had, what, four glasses already, judging by the bill, which I've just picked up.

'How will you get there at this time of night?'

'Oh, I'm driving.'

'No, seriously, Izz, you can't drive. I won't let you. And when in God's name did you pass your test?'

She leans, wobbles, whispers. 'I didn't! C'mon, you want to come too?'

There is no way I am getting in a car with her, and there is no way I am letting her drive.

'Have you got a fiver, for a tip?' I ask her. She opens her bag, and like a whippet I dive in, grab her car keys and stuff them down my bra.

'I am not letting you get in that car,' I tell her. 'I am ordering you an Uber.'

LIZ JONES

CHAPTER SIX
I'm a sponge

I have one last try to thin myself manually. Months
ago, Izzy had sent me an email asking whether I wanted
to do the Camberwell 10k with her in aid of Cancer
Research. I said yes, after first asking whether or not
it was hilly, thinking if I increased from a puffy crawl
to a walk to a brisk walk to a jog in increments of five
steps a day I'd be ready by then. Problem is, I forgot
all about it.

And then, yesterday, she warned me it's tomorrow.
Oh Jesus Christ. I have no idea where my trainers are.
Or my sports bra. Or my black leggings. Oh, there they
are, at the bottom of the laundry basket. Oh dear, they
still have a pair of knickers attached from when I last
peeled them off after an ill-fated egg and spoon.

I meet her at the start, just near the green. There
are far more women than men milling around in jazzy
leggings and tight crop tops, sucking on water bottles
like lambs on the teat. I haven't brought any water

99

as I hadn't planned on putting on that much speed; also I may hail a taxi halfway round. I have a sweatshirt knotted round my middle, to hide various parts of my anatomy I don't want people watching jogging up and down. I know it's supposed to be a fun run, but I don't want to encourage quite that level of hilarity.

While Izzy fetches our numbers, I watch everyone getting ready, chatting, having their calves massaged. The women are all shapes, ages and sizes, when I had thought everyone would resemble Dame Kelly Holmes. It's quite a touching scene, really, so strangely moving that I feel a bit tearful. Every single woman is trying to improve herself. They are all doing their best. For a man, probably. Never mind the gender pay gap, upskirting, the glass ceiling and the loudly ticking biological clock. My belief is the way men and women prepare for dates is the biggest obstacle (oh dear God, there won't be jumps, will there? This isn't like the cross-country run at Brentwood High, is it, when I refused the water jump, like a donkey faced with Becher's Brook at the Grand National?) we face in the fight for equality.

Take Izzy, who has a hot date planned for tomorrow night: she has had her roots retouched, has read the man's latest book so she can chat to him about it, measured the distance between her house and his chosen venue using a little wheelie thing to see if it's doable in heels, changed her sheets, bought a new dress and underwear and now she is about to huff and puff over the course of six miles while holding onto her breasts ('Too expensive to risk too much movement') to make up for the fact she will doubtless have to eat dinner with him so he doesn't think her high-maintenance and odd.

Men, on the other hand, are not here to impress women. They are here to beat other men, or themselves, given the number of times they glance at their Apple watches and press little buttons. They are not getting fit or trying to lose weight for *us*.

We set off. It's fine. This is easy! I don't know why people make so much fuss! I think from now on I will go for a run at 6 a.m. every day before coming back home for a green smoothie! Who needs an expensive operation when I can run for free! Izzy is clasping onto both breasts. I tell her she should be more worried about her face dropping, which is apparently what happens if women run too much; maybe there is some sort of sling she can wear on her head.

'Don't make me laugh,' she says. 'I will wet myself. Anyway, it's not my face I'm worried about, it's my arse!'

As she, as well as the entire entry, is now in front of me, I take a good look at it. It is perfectly spherical. Exactly the right size, whatever the right size is. She is worried about getting an 'African bum', as she calls it, just like her mum's.

I'm a bit hot now. I know my face is fluorescent pink, I can just feel it. I wonder how much further. I wish I had brought water. I have to unwrap the sweatshirt and carry it in a small bundle. I have just been overtaken by two army cadets, who are walking. There are snails who are faster than me. There are straggled lines of onlookers, clapping, cheering us on. When I run (who am I kidding? When I shuffle) past them, one woman says, 'Are you alright, love?'

'Yes,' I hiss, not wanting to waste oxygen. 'Bit of a tight Achilles.'

A small boy actually laughs.

I give up. I stop and lean my hands on my knees. I spy an M&S in the distance, shimmering like a mirage. I wonder if I can just pop in there, get a bottle of water. Lucozade. A sausage roll. An Uber electric bike. My nipples are sore.

I do complete the fun run, though it wasn't fun, and more of a walk really. I am dripping with sweat. As I near the end, the clapping and cheering spurs me on a bit, so I do cross the finish line and take delivery of my T-shirt and medal to prove I did it. But I cannot imagine ever doing it again. Izzy is waiting, camera poised to take a photo. She hands me a bottle of water. I look for somewhere to sit down. I really want an ice cream. This is too hard. This will take years.

The next day, I get a text. 'Hi, Pamela. Thank you for completing the Camberwell 10k run. Your position is 2,250th, your personal time is 02.23.25, your gun time is 02.23.36. Please send monies raised to …'

I'm given the details of a bank account. Oh dear. I was so busy navel-gazing – literally – I forgot to raise any money!

. . .

And so it is that I am all alone in the small, pristine hospital room. I'm sat on the bed, in a gown that is rather worryingly open at the back; I can actually feel the Gulf Stream. I've had nothing to eat since last night, so am starving. I had to break it to Neps I was having surgery, as I think he might have noticed my absence for at least a week, if not two. I lied about how much it was going to cost: told him it was a freebie. Once I wake up tomorrow, the plan is for him to come and collect me in a taxi so I can recuperate at home and be fed pineapple juice (helps reduce swelling holistically) via a straw. I've been told I won't be able to drive, or lift anything, or sneeze, or put things in washing machines for four weeks. It will be like a little holiday, surely?

And here's the thing. Neps wasn't even that concerned when I gravely broke the news to him. He didn't try to talk me out of it. He didn't say, well, you don't need surgery, you are lovely just as you are. He merely wondered if I could possibly line up a week's worth of packed lunches for the twins in the fridge and could he borrow my phone charger.

And here's another thing: he didn't even bring me here. I had to take an Uber. 'It's not as if you're ill,' he said. 'This is your choice. Don't rope me into your self-obsessed paranoia.'

Charming. I could have said, well, it's not my choice when it came to who my parents were. It's not my choice that we happened to have twins, which was as much your fault as mine. (Everyone assumes we used IVF, and a turkey baster, but that is absolutely not the case. It turns out twins run in his family, something he had failed to point out before he impregnated me; if I'd known, I'd have beaten him off with a wooden spoon.) It is not my choice to be this unhappy, this abnormal. At least I am trying to do something about the way I look and about my health. Get promoted, perhaps. And do something about my ability to be a good wife to him. To make him happy and proud. And aroused.

There is a soft knock on the door. Ooh, drugs.

It turns out to be a young man, sent by the surgeon's PR, who is going to take before and after photos. This is the price I have to pay for getting such a huge discount. The photos will be posted on the surgeon's website, along with my diary of my surgery. I'd glossed over the fact this was happening, hoping, as I usually do, that everyone would forget about it and it would never, ever happen. But no. Here he is. A bearded hipster in combat gear. I feel moved to ask, 'Where's the war?'

'So,' he says, 'I think I met your husband once, at a party.'

'Oh, really?' I can tell he is not in the least bit interested in me and that his true ambition in life is to photograph Bella Hadid naked. He hasn't even learned my name. 'Do you want to take the photo now?' I ask him, hoping that then he will go.

'No rush. Maybe I could order something to drink?'

'It's not a hotel.'

'No, but it is private, isn't it?'

It turns out he needs a photo of my Before Stomach, front, side and back, with me just wearing my pants. 'I can cut your head off,' he says helpfully. He will return in a couple of months to take the After Stomach; if the desired effect isn't good enough, he says, failing to be very encouraging at all, he can 'always airbrush' me.

Just as I am taking my robe off and sliding from the table, like lava down Mount Etna, Jasmine enters. The weather changes when Jasmine enters a room: the sun shines, birds sing, flower buds unfurl, salmon leap, meerkats sit up straight. The photographer perks up. Jasmine immediately susses the situation and tells him,

Hattie Jacques-fashion, 'You will have to be quick! We are going to take the lift down to the operating theatre now!'

'I'll come with you,' he says.

I am pretty fed up, to be honest, always being the least attractive person in the room. Other people are never scared of you, or interested in you, when you are fat. At a meeting, because you are deemed the least attractive person in the room – despite the bald men, the buck-toothed, cross-eyed women with boils on their noses and nervous tics – you are always the one dispatched to fetch an easel or lattes. You are never a threat when it comes to snaring men, a great job, the best deckchair: people assume you will simply go straight through and land on the floor. In a weird way, I think this is why I've succeeded, a little bit, at being a PR. Forced to be backstage at a fashion show to make sure everything runs smoothly and no one overdoses, the models and stylists don't see me as a rival, or as someone they need to impress, so they confide in me and tell me things. I'm just furniture, or a sponge. I'm big, so I must be cuddly. I'm big, so I can't possibly have an ego, or feelings. Even when I'm the one having a dangerous procedure, even though I'm the reason the stupid trendy man is here on a Saturday probably earning double time, now the pretty nurse has arrived I'm suddenly just a squashy armchair in the corner of the room.

We are in the lift, we strange threesome. I can sense the photographer is enjoying being so close to Jasmine. I wonder what it feels like, being her. I wonder if she sails through life, given her green eyes, her black hair, her tiny waist and non-existent breasts. What problems could you possibly have if you look like that? No one would care what you wore, or where you lived, or what you drove, or how intelligent you were. They would just gaze at you. You wouldn't even have to say anything. You would never have to pay for anything, I'm positive of that. You would never have to demand anything, stamp your feet, cheep like a parrot. It would all just come to you, as easy as a flower welcoming a hungry drone.

As we descend to the basement I suddenly notice, much to my extreme horror, that my bare arse is being reflected in the shiny walls of the lift behind me. A huge, flat moon of chubbiness above two stubby thighs. I gasp, shocked, ashamed, until I realise no one else is looking at the wall. Only me. Bearded Hipster and Gorgeous Nurse only have eyes for each other. As I gaze at the image, I realise I'd been so fixated on my stomach and the flap I had forgotten what disaster was going on out back. And I begin to wonder where the plastic surgery will end: will I become the Forth Bridge, or a magician trying to keep plates afloat on top of sticks: fixing one bit, then hurrying onto the next before everything smashes to the floor? As I look at my arse, reflected in the lift, I can't help but smile at the irony of the likes of Kim Kardashian being held up as a bigger role model. Kim Kardashian and Jennifer Lopez and Beyoncé are no nearer to what I resemble naked than Kate Moss or Karlie Kloss. The only time I have ever seen someone who remotely looks like me naked in the media was when Alexander McQueen's Spring/Summer 2001 Voss show was reviewed, and in order to disentangle his inspiration, magazines were forced to reproduce the shocking and hideous photograph by Joel-Peter Witkin: an obese woman, her face concealed by an antiquated oxygen mask, imprisoned in an asylum. Which pretty much sums me up.

Jasmine is now staring at me, making sure I'm okay. I give her a watery smile.

Finally, we emerge (I attempt to go last, because of the exposed-to-the-elements arse, but unfortunately Jasmine ushers me to go first; I end up creeping sideways like a giant crab) and I am shown into the operating theatre's anteroom. I clamber onto yet another table covered in paper and all the rustling as I heave my bulk suddenly reminds me incongruously of Mum's cakes: little stiff collars of greaseproof or a disc stuck to the bottom, or a nest in a biscuit tin. And I realise all that food wasn't worth it now I've had to sit with a bare arse in an operating theatre. How much joy was in each bite, really, before it turned to regret and guilt? How much washing-up was there to do afterwards, as well as supermarket shopping, and lugging, and sit-ups, and the treadmill, and trying to jog up Primrose Hill before being towed by a passing – and, as it turned out, stoic and patient – yellow Lab.

I notice a list of patients on the wall. The name, procedure and then a tick by the side; no deaths so far. Phew. Always a plus. I am last on the list, after three men, each of whom has had liposuction. So, it is not just women who suffer from cellulite and self-doubt, after all. Men just hide it better. Who'd have thought.

I lie back and a needle is placed in my arm by someone who tells me he is the anaesthetist: I can see crinkly kind eyes above a green surgical mask. I expected judgement, but there is none. I am asked to count backwards from 50. More bleeding homework. It was bad enough reading all my post-op instructions. I reach 47 and then it is over. I know no more. I can no longer hear the camera whirring and clicking. I slip into oblivion. When I wake, I will be thin. I will be reborn. My life will start.

8$^1/_2$ STONE

PART 2
LITTLE PAM'S STORY

$8\frac{1}{2}$ STONE

CHAPTER SEVEN
I must ring Norris and Ross McWhirter

I can't open my eyes. They seem glued shut. I try to move my arm, to feel what is happening to my face, but some sort of tube makes it spring back, keeps it tethered. I can hear people talking. Ah, so I'm not brain-dead: a cabbage or a kale. That's something, I suppose. I let out a noise, a sort of moan. A hand touches my other arm.

'Are you awake, my darling? Now, don't move. Just let me remove the tape from your lids, then I will get you some water.'

There is some slow unplastering, which feels as though my eyelashes are being waxed. The light is very bright indeed. I open my eyes. I see huge strip lights above me. I am on a trolley, and I am still in the anteroom. My mouth is dry. I try to form words.

'Wha appen. Di you no do i? Di you no cut i ow!'

Jasmine. At last, a friendly face.

'No, don't worry. We were just waiting for you to come round properly before we take you back to your room. It all went very well. The tuck is very neat, I've seen it, I was with you the whole time. You have a dressing on it. And some drains from your abdomen, which will feel odd, but they will come out tomorrow. Try not to move too much. I can sit you up a little. Oooof. Let me know if you feel faint at any point.'

. . .

I am now sitting up in bed, back in my safe little room. At first, it wasn't too bad. I must have been pumped full of drugs. Seven hours later and I'm in complete agony. It hurts to breathe. I am so swollen I am bigger than I was before the surgery, which has sent me into even more of a decline. Apparently, during liposuction the surgeon removed seven pounds of fat. Seven pounds! That's nothing! I poo more than that in one sitting! The bag, though, Jasmine assured me, is gone. There is a nice, neat seam, like something on a Kirstie Allsopp Handmade Christmas programme. I can't see this, though, as I am swaddled in bandages.

I was expecting flowers in my room. I know I haven't had a baby, but I have expelled roughly the same amount as one small infant, or half a twin. I was also expecting Neps to be there, perhaps reading his huge tome in a corner of the room. But no, there is no one. Even the Taliban fighting photographer has gone, probably to a warehouse party, or off on a mini-break, while I am prone on a narrow bed, silently screaming. I am only to spend one night here, before Neps comes to pick me up to reduce costs. But I don't feel remotely ready. I start to panic. I would hyperventilate if I could, but it hurts too much to breathe.

There are no messages or missed calls on my phone. And so, I break the habit of a lifetime and I call him. As I do so, I notice my wedding band and engagement ring have been removed; they were worried about infection, of course, and my earrings have gone as well, but in my current state of mind it feels like an Ominous Sign. It is late, I expect the twins are in bed and of course he will be, too, but I don't care. I am his wife. I have rights. If not conjugal ones.

It rings and rings and rings. And rings. And rings.

Finally. He picks up. He sounds groggy.

'Who is this?'

'What do you mean, who is this? It's your wife! Just come round from life-threatening surgery?'

'Oh, yeah, sorry, I was asleep. [He actually yawns. I really hate people who yawn. It is passive aggressive.] I've had a really difficult day. I did call the hospital earlier, but they said you were still under.'

'Well, I'm not now. I am very much wide awake!'

'I can come and visit you tomorrow afternoon.

The twins have school and so do I.'

'I won't be here tomorrow, remember. You are coming to pick me up.' I bet he wishes it were just a visit, before he could escape again, out into a world of exciting possibilities.

'Oh, yeah. I forgot.'

'Can you call and ask them to bring me some food? I've been pressing a buzzer, but I think it was the wrong one, the one for painkiller, because I'm now feeling a bit odd.'

'Yeah, okay. What do you want?'

'Oh, anything. Pineapple. A cheeseburger. I'm starving. I was nil by mouth last night, remember, and now they won't bring room service.'

'Okay.'

'Aren't you going to ask how I am?'

'Yes, I was going to, but you didn't give me a chance. How are you?'

'Not great, to be honest, I'm in a great deal of pain.'

'Press the button some more. Look, I really have to go. I will call you in the morning.'

He has pressed 'End' before I've even had a chance to respond. I stare at the phone, suddenly inert in my hands. I can't believe he just did that. It's as though I am nothing. An annoyance. A splinter; well, a thorn, at least until the swelling goes down. I'm angry, to be honest, and a bit shocked. This is akin to childbirth, all over again. I'm not sure if I'm imagining it, but he sounded odd. The air around him seemed thick, charged. And he couldn't wait to put the phone down. Which is a cheek, as I am doing this FOR HIM!

. . .

An hour later and I am doubled up in pain. Well, not quite doubled, as there is too much flesh and fluid, but sort of scrunched up in pain, like a punctured football. The food arrived, but I couldn't face it. That must be something of a world record: I must ring Norris and Ross McWhirter. It is very late now and there doesn't seem to be anyone on duty, as no one has popped their head round the door, or checked my drip or my drain, or looked at my chart, or come to ask me how I am. I am sure something has gone wrong. I feel nauseous, but I cannot allow myself to be sick, as it would be far too painful. It still hurts to breathe, so I just take small little pants. This thought reminds me why I had surgery in the first place. I'm suddenly hopeful. I will be able to wear small little pants.

I am desperate to go to the loo, and to move, and so I manage to lift the sheet – ow! – off me and swing my legs over the side. My top half is still lying down, but I can't sit up, so I sort of roll over onto my side – oof! – managing to pull out the drip and the drain in the process. Oh no. Perhaps I shouldn't have done this; I should have just rung Neps again, told him to get a kidney dish sent up. But on second thoughts, no. I don't want him to think me less attractive than he already does. My feet and calves are encased in thick white pop socks; what is this, the seventies? I am still wearing the stupid gown. I manage to shuffle to my en suite on my bottom. Finally, after what seems an age, I am by the loo and I manage to hoist myself up, turn on the light with the cord thing and lower my bruised bulk. The relief is immense.

I get up, lean on the sink and go to wash my hands. I look up, breaking the habit of a lifetime, and see my face staring back at me. Gahhh! Why is my face bruised? Swollen? Why am I bigger than I was before?

And then it hits me. A rounders ball smack bang in the face. What have I done? I have made myself worse than I was before! I now have scars everywhere. I haven't seen them, as they are lurking beneath the bandages, waiting to spring out and upset me, but I know they are there, waiting like grotesque, livid tattoos (they're livid; try being me!), done while drunk, inking the name of a man I think I will love forever on my skin before finding out he's run off with the woman from Costa Coffee. I will never be able to have more children: the surgeon said as much. I now have no money. My husband still isn't interested in me. And I start to cry, huge heaving sobs that hurt and pull at every stitch. I am ruined. Why on earth did I do this to myself? I'm a laughing stock in pop socks.

I can't think clearly, which I think is the drugs, but there is a voice, in the distance, whispering that I should kill myself. I have heard this voice before, you know, but I have never acted on it. The first time was when I was a child – I must have been very young – in bed, hearing my parents shouting; I just didn't want to be there. Because what is the point, life being this hard? No one cares about me. No one cares if I am gone. There is a voice, telling me that my family will be better off without me: I am so flawed, so incomplete, so not in control of anything. He will be able to marry someone else, someone thin, someone who can have children with him. Someone who will come first in the egg and spoon.

I look around for something to use. I see my leggings, draped, tent-fashion, on the chair; Christo could cover buildings with these – I must remember to email him, suggest my giant pants be upcycled after I'm gone. I try to make them into a rope and sling them over the shower rail – ow! Dear God that hurt. I put the legs round my neck – oh God the pain, I want it to stop. I knot it, like a scarf. I can't climb on anything, so I decide to sink to the floor. It happens slowly; it tightens a little, but then my great big bulk pulls the railing from the wall.

119

I'm sure I also now have a head injury.

I am so completely useless. I can't even perform the simplest task. There must be something else I can do to end my stupid life. Throw myself in front of a train? No, I won't get far in my nightie. Ah! I know! I find my pink Ladyshave and decide to stab at my wrists, but nothing happens. I don't even draw blood. Frustrated, desperate, I throw the stupid thing at the mirror, which doesn't even shatter.

I have to find someone to help me. I must be allergic to something, as I am starting to feel strange. I feel such shame that I want to end it all: I'm a mum, for Christ's sake. I have responsibilities. I think I just want someone to feel sorry for me. I feel I have to get out, escape, find help, and so I stagger from the room, holding onto the walls. I find a lift, the one we used before, when I was WHOLE. I step in, avoiding my reflection this time, and I press G. There must be someone on reception. Why is there no one around? It's not an NHS hospital, for Christ's sake! It's not Syria!

The lift lands and the jolt makes me cry out. I crawl on my hands and knees. Help! Help! I am still holding onto walls and chairs. A red stain has appeared on my stomach. Oh no! I must have burst some of the stitches. There is blood everywhere.

There is an arched door and I press it and go in.

Ah, it's a chapel. Presumably where people who have lost loved ones, or been told they have cancer, go to pray. Why was I so stupid? There was nothing wrong with me! Even Izzy hasn't texted, and this was partly or mostly her fault!

At last, somewhere to sit. I slide into a bench. Oh, now that's a surprise. For the first time, I can fit into a pew. Maybe it did work. Just a little. Oh God, all I wanted was to be thin. To be normal. To be eight and a half stone. Was that too much to ask? Am I being punished for being so vain?

. . .

The next morning, I'm feeling a tiny bit better. I can burp without screaming. Always a plus. I've had a cup of tea. Jasmine says I look brighter, that everyone feels suicidal the night after surgery: everyone thinks cosmetic surgery is the easy option, a cop-out, when it's the opposite, even harder and more painful than a 10k run. She tells me not to be discouraged. I still look big because I am swollen and I will deflate nicely in a few days. I need to drink lots of water and presumably eat lots of pineapples.

Neps is coming to pick me up today, once he's dropped the twins off at school. He hasn't phoned, but he has sent a couple of texts.

'Hi. Hope you are well. Will be there at 11 a.m. Do

121

you know where the key is for the gas meter?'

I'm like his maiden aunt, seriously.

And another one, which must be something of a record. I sometimes think men believe they have a finite number of texts allotted before they die and hence don't want to waste one. 'Hi. Found it. On my way.'

I am dressed, thanks to Jasmine, who I am sure will make a very good mum one day, and am sat on the edge of the bed with my holdall, exactly like a refugee after a shipwreck, my mouth in a wounded Charlie Brown zigzag, when he finally turns up, 20 minutes late. He doesn't really look at me: his eyes seem unable to land on my form. I struggle to get off the bed, but he doesn't move to help me, just grabs my bag, says, 'Have you left anything in the bathroom?' He thinks I brought this on myself. He told me not to do it – at the eleventh hour he mumbled something about how he would help more, so I had more time to go to the gym and cook from scratch, which all sounded like more hard work for me! – and I didn't listen. At the time, I felt I had no choice. Nothing worked: not the diets, not my marriage. My big bulk, the tummy flap, were getting in the way of everything. I'd had to be brave, to do this, but now my courage is seeping out of me, just like the watery stuff on the bandages. I'm wondering if I've made a huge mistake.

Jasmine arrives to say goodbye. She ignores Neps

pointedly, and gingerly takes an elbow: the only small bit of me that doesn't hurt. She has a stiff paper bag full of painkillers and antibiotics, which she hands wordlessly to him. I can tell by her body language she disapproves of him, and I am so grateful to have someone who is on my side I am finding it hard to leave her. What does she see that I don't?

We are in a black cab, after lots of ouches and aargghs. Every time a speed bump hoves into view, I grimace at Neps. 'Tell the driver to slow down!' I beg of him. But he refuses. He is, of course, on the side of the poor put-upon taxi driver, not his wife and the mother of his children, who has gone under the knife to be cured of her extreme fatness, when so many people in the world do not have enough to eat. Oh yes. I do know I am the bad person. That his brownness trumps my pinkness every single time.

After an age, we are finally outside our little house. Neps pays, ostentatiously adding a generous tip: a scrunched-up fiver, just to show how material things mean nothing to him. 'Thanks, mate,' he says, giving the driver the full wattage of his teeth. Oh, that he smiled at me like that. He helps me inside the house. I've only been gone just over 24 hours but everything seems different. Flat. Empty. He helps me up the stairs, drops my bag in the room. 'Blimey!' I say. 'You've changed the sheets!'

This is something of a miracle. When Neps and his

collection of trainers and hip-hop CDs first moved in, he hadn't even known duvets have covers.

'Of course I have. Clean towels. Got some shopping in. I'm not entirely useless, you know.'

He leaves me then; I know he has reluctantly taken a day off work, so I should be grateful, but somehow I just can't rally the emotion. I don't bother to undress, I just get into bed, unable to bear even the weight of the duvet on my tummy. I close my eyes, and a few minutes later hear him come into the room. 'Here,' he says, handing me a plastic punnet of grapes. They haven't even been washed, while a bowl was clearly too much bother. I notice the skeleton of a long-dead spider wedged between two wrinkled purple globes.

CHAPTER EIGHT

I find out there's a reason he's turned into Captain Haddock

Three months later

The scar is still red, and angry, like a rictus Jack Nicholson grin in my knicker line, but the flap is gone, hurrah! I'd have liked to have kept it, really, in a glass jar, preserved in formaldehyde. As a hideous warning against Western consumerism, greed and two-for-one offers. Or donated it to science, so that medical students could learn about the dangers of yo-yo dieting, Twixes and reading Vogue. The bruising from the lipo, which fascinated me for a while, changing from purple to green to yellow, has vanished and, as promised, I have deflated somewhat. The only evidence I have of being vacuumed are four tiny red dots. In front of me on the bed is a pair of jeans: a gauntlet of gauntness.

My size-16 skinny jeans.

They lie, inky and unworn. A vessel containing my

hopes and dreams and, hopefully, today and for the very first time, my arse.

I have chosen a quiet time to do this little exercise. It's a Saturday. The twins are at swimming, Neps is at the gym (Sainsbury's would have been more useful, but at least he's out of the house) and so I have the place to myself. Aside from the cat, who is regarding me from the top of the chest of drawers with an expression that says, 'I can now fit through the cat flap, thanks to those dreaded diet biscuits. Now, let's see if you can do it, too.'

I am feeling hopeful, buoyant even, that I will be able to get into them. Excited. A slightly counter-intuitive state to be in, I have to admit, given the horror that has been the last three months. Never mind the surgery, the pain, the nausea, the suicidal thoughts, the stitches, the expense, the time off work, the disapproval from him, from my mum, the pain – or did I already mention that? I have been too confused, too scared, too upset to even think about eating. The fat bird in me whispers in my ear: who knew that misery was such a great friend to becoming a stick insect? We should have tried it out before! They should wheel out cheating husbands on the NHS, be a whole lot cheaper than treating all those diabetes patients with drugs. Cuckolding and betrayal instead of wiring up your jaw or stapling your stomach.

But it has been as though I am schizophrenic. (Is

it okay to call it this? Or should I say bipolar?) As the horror of everything that's happened since the op unfolded, and the weeks limped by, and I felt too miserable, too stupid and blind to reality to eat, I couldn't help but look at my arse in the mirror in the bathroom, twisting this way and that before experiencing a tiny frisson of joy. I deliberately enter Selfridges through the revolving doors at the front, rather than skulk in through a side entrance. Gliding up the escalators, I even pose like a mannequin, alighting at Women's Designer Wear, running a thin(ner) hand along the rails, not even bothering to peer at the sizes to see if they have mine. Of course they have mine. I am normal. I am almost sample size. My God. I always used to hate women like me.

. . .

I'm thin(ner) now. Why can't everything be easy!?

To be honest, I don't know where to start. I'm so ashamed to have to type this. But maybe typing it will make it more bearable; I once had a therapist who told me to write down my problems on a piece of paper, fold the paper up and place it in an envelope, then a drawer, and then to lock it. The problem is still there, but it is removed. It can no longer hurt you. So. Okay. Here we go.

I think it was me being vulnerable, more dependent

than usual that caused the mask and the pretence (and the boxer shorts) to slip. Or maybe he was simply exhausted from not just looking after me but the twins and the cat as well that he forgot to lie, cover his tracks. It turns out it's true, that cliché about men being unable to multitask; I'd always thought it an excuse so they could get out of doing things. He couldn't be truly present, be a husband and a dad, load the dishwasher, arrange his features into something that approximated sympathy and conduct an affair. It was all too much. Something had to give and for once it wasn't my waistband.

It was the small things at first that set off tiny alarms I refused to listen to. Such as on that first day home after surgery, the one with the unwashed grapes, when I went to reach for the glass of water on the bedside table and noticed it was just out of reach. Why would he move the furniture? He never moves furniture. To him, such lowly things as a chair or a table don't even exist. The lampshade on my side of the bed was at a funny angle. But. I don't know. Maybe he knocked it when he changed the linen.

Then there was the fact he kept looking at his phone, even more frequently than usual. Even when answering a question from me or the kids, his eyes would be looking at his screen. Refresh. Refresh. Refresh. Then, he would get a text and his face would light up. A smile would crease one side of his face;

he would push it down, but it would bob right back up again, like those gas canisters they attached to Jaws. Whoosh, whoosh, whoosh. After a week or two when I told him, listen, I won't break, I need a cuddle, he put both hands in the air as if to show he was unarmed and said, 'Look. I don't really want to go there. Then be blamed for hurting you.'

'As if you could hurt me,' I said.

Women don't really need hard evidence of betrayal, because we always feel it, like a draught from an open window. We can tell from the angle of an eyebrow. The first time I was able to come down to the kitchen, after two days in bed, he looked up, mid-making himself a smoothie, and his face said it all. Oh no. She's mobile again. She's on the move! She's invading my space. It was the angles of his face that said it. The slope of his shoulders. His breathing. When I came into view in my blue nightie, it was as though he had just received a letter from the Home Secretary saying, 'Sorry, mate, the sentence has not been revoked. You are still married. You will still be hung at dawn as planned. Now, what do you want in your last smoothie?'

Half-term, and although I had a check-up booked with the surgeon, when I would be measured and weighed, he said he couldn't come with me. It's important, so why on earth not?

'I'm meeting a poet. She's an amAZing writer. From

Kolkata.'

I could tell by the exaggerated way he pronounced the name of India's cultural hotbed, along with a little head shake, that he was resentful of me, what with my first-world problems and idiotic job.

'Oh really? That's nice. What's her name?'

'You won't have heard of her.'

'I know, but I can look her up. I'm interested. Where are you meeting her?'

'Islington. She's staying with some friends.'

I wish I were the sort of person who stays with friends. Whenever I go anywhere, I always have to endure a Premier Inn and pay extra for Wi-Fi and parking. I am always asked to hand over my credit card so that it can be 'pre-authorised'; a modern method of stealing.

So as not to appear secretive, he went on, 'I'm asking if she has time to come down to the school, inspire my class.'

'But they're all on holiday.' (Free to roam the streets stabbing people, more like.)

'I know that. When they get back next week. I'm just sounding her out.'

He finally told me her name – he couldn't help a smirk as the delicious consonants and vowels of her name passed over his tongue – before he set off, his wide shoulders in a navy sweater, narrow hips in white jeans I'd not seen before. Loafers. No socks. (That is new, the no socks thing. Creates less washing, I suppose.) As soon as I heard the door slam, I typed her name frantically into my phone before I forgot it. I searched for photos and there she was. A vision. Young, with thick eyebrows, beautiful. Accomplished, the winner of numerous new young writer awards. Bit of a low forehead but she's young, you see. Did I tell you that? It turned out she was in town for a literary festival in Bloomsbury: the theme was diversity, nature and emerging talent. I imagine her coffee-coloured tummy is untrammelled, perfect, flat. It doesn't have little white railway tracks where the stitches once were.

And so. I decided to follow him.

Well, not exactly follow him, as I don't inhabit a spy movie, but, having exposed my scars to Mr Kalimares and got the all-clear, and been told I'm 'doing really well' and 'don't forget, I am offering 10 per cent off our Learn to Love Your Pins Lipo', I decided to turn up that evening at her 'event', which was already creating quite a buzz on Facebook. I called Izzy. At first, she thought I'd gone mad.

'But look at how much weight you've lost! You're so much slimmer and, yeah, okay, she's a poet, an artist really, I have heard of her, gorgeous, I think she was a Bollywood star before she found her brain, but then you are so funny,' she said, as if that would be any defence against a dark-eyed beauty from his motherland. It would be like a Miss World contest between Arundhati Roy and Pam Ayres.

'Will you come with me?' I pleaded. 'I can hide at the back and you can chat to her, put your PR hat on over your headscarf. Come on, I know something is up. She is just his type. Clever. Pure. Thin but not Western thin.'

She finally agreed. I dropped the twins off at Mum's and picked her up in an Uber.

She slid into the seat next to me, tossing her mane of glossy black hair. The driver immediately angled his rear mirror to look at her. They never, ever do that with me: another of life's small slights. 'This is quite exciting!' she said, depositing her phone in her huge tote, crossing her long limbs before gesturing at the driver to keep his eyes on the road.

'Now, listen to me,' I said, suddenly Mrs Richards from Fawlty Towers. Dear God, no wonder he's panting after Priyanka Chopra. 'He can't see me, so it is all down to you. He might not even be there. He might well have met her, told her about the kids at his school who can't use utensils let alone grasp poetry, and be on his way home. I just need to reassure myself before I start throwing accusations and plates.'

'Yeah. I'm sure she's already deeply unhappy in an arranged marriage,' she said loyally.

We headed north across the river. Everything seemed

normal. Buses. People hurrying along, heads down, looking at their phones. Seagulls. My world won't end surely when there are still black cabs in the world and cyclists swearing. My goodness, everything looks better seen through thin eyes. (It's strange, that I can no longer see my cheeks in the periphery of my vision. I'm smaller, but the world is suddenly bigger.)

We pulled up at a huge white Art Deco building on one side of Bloomsbury Square. I remember I'd been to a fashion launch here once and I suddenly felt nostalgic for my old life, BCE: Before Cunting Excision. We disembarked and as it all became more real I felt silly for having brought her here. For mistrusting him. The problem, you see, is my complete lack of self-esteem, not his rampant libido. A placard, bearing a large photo of the Trollop, pointed the way down some stone steps; I made Izzy lead the way. My stomach and thighs still hurt, which meant I couldn't yet manage heels, so I was in ballet flats. As we neared the auditorium, I felt short and lumpen. Impossibly unattractive. Who could blame him, frankly, falling for a dark-haired temptress who pens poems rather than press releases?

There was the loud buzz of talking: it had the slightly hysterical air of young people who think they are 'where it's at': i.e. the centre of the cultural and intellectual universe, while the rest of us are waiting for Emmerdale to start. I lurked at the back, while Izzy strode towards the stage. She'd dug out her phone and opened the camera: 'For evidence,' she hissed.

There were rows of chairs, lots of women in saris and men with beards. Oh, did I tell you Neps had been growing his beard since a few days before I had surgery? He knows I hate it; I'm always frightened he'll be shot by the police, or at the very least tasered, but he persisted anyway. He would have fed it from a watering can each morning if he could, like a tomato plant. The beard made him feel even more of a stranger in the house.

At the end of the room was a table, flanked by two low chairs and holding a carafe of water, two glasses and microphones. I suddenly saw her, the poet. The Whore. She was hard to miss. She was in a gold and blue sari, which exposed a delicious sliver of dark, taut skin. Even from here I could see she had huge dark eyes, a full mouth. She was animated, confident, smiling. Damn! I thought. Damn! No amount of surgery could turn me into that. My body would have to be melted down, like Morph, and everything started again from scratch to achieve what she has.

I could see Izzy, pretending to text near the stage, having pulled her scarf over her head, keeping one eye on the temptress. And then, at the edge of my vision, I was aware of a shape, an aura, as familiar to me as my own reflection, or my own children. It was Neps, but also not Neps. It was him, but he was almost bouncing on his toes, like a boxer before a prize fight. He no longer seemed rooted to the spot, but free. Upright. Inches taller. Engaged. Oh, dear Lord, he's not asked her to marry him already, has he?

While I hid behind a plant, he busied about a bit, put something in his manbag and then leaned across the table, next to which was the poet, who was probably rearranging her thong, and another man: a white man I hadn't noticed until just now. This man also had a beard; it must be catching. I remember thinking, as I saw the scene unfold to my horror in slow motion, I bet that beard's ginger in some lights. The poet meanwhile seemed disinterested in Neps and so I started to relax a little. Phew.

But I spoke too soon. Suddenly the ginger beard and Neps's Captain Haddock black growth locked and their lips landed on each other. They stayed like that for several seconds – so long, in fact, I thought their beards might be acting like Velcro, cementing them in an unwilling embrace. But no. Finally, they parted. They smiled. Neps actually then touched the ginger man's face with the back of one slow, affectionate hand. It was like that moment between Patrick Swayze and Jennifer Grey all over again. I could feel the warmth between them from the back of the 'space'.

. . .

What happened next is all a bit of a blur. Izzy belatedly realised what was happening. I saw her shocked face turn towards me. Neps spotted her, walked over to say hello, perhaps do a bit of firefighting, or, as I like to call it, lying through his teeth, but then reality dawned, and he turned reluctantly and saw me lurking at the back of the 'space': a blob of hurt pinkness, a weight around his feet and his desire. Thing is, though, he didn't wave or come striding towards me, professing his love and his innocence. He carried on chatting, to other people, to the poet. He even slapped Ginger Man on the back, made a gesture that meant 'laters', and disappeared out a back entrance. Even that was odd. Your wife sees you snogging another man and you ignore her. But then, I always knew he was a coward.

Izzy, scarf and gloves off, strode towards me, helped me up the steps, which for the first time in my adult life I was finding relatively easy – my goodness, moving through space is a breeze when you're not carrying another adult human being about your person – and we hailed a cab. Or wailed a cab, given I was sobbing.

'What just happened?' she asked me.

'I don't know,' I said between gulps. 'Well, I do know. I think I've always known. No man is that distracted, surely.'

'But is he gay?' she asked sweetly.

'Maybe. Maybe he couldn't bear to tell his parents. You know what they're like. I always felt more like his mum than his wife. Maybe it wasn't the fat or the flap or the stretch marks that turned him off, it was the fact I own a vagina.'

She almost laughed, then put her head on one side. 'Well, you know what? At least you know now it's not your fault he's been so strange.'

'But what do I do now? Will he be at home? Do I have to buy a strap-on?'

'Where else has he got to go?' she said, peering out the window, as if trying to spot him. 'His parents won't want him: they will go mad when they find out he's cheated on you! Especially with a man! He has children!'

'I know that!' I almost snapped. 'I'm sorry. It's still a shock, even though I knew something wasn't right. I mean, what straight man irons tea towels?'

'Do you want me to come home with you? Wait till he's back?'

'No. But can you get the twins from Mum, have them at yours? So that we can argue properly? Please don't take coke in front of them. Is your E in a locked cupboard?'

'Okay, yes, I promise. No rolled bank notes or mirrors. I'll look after them, don't worry. You do what you have to do.'

8½ STONE

CHAPTER NINE

Let her cardis be snagged
for the next six months

And that was it. That was how I lost the rest of the weight and am here, now, staring at my skinny jeans, the only good thing, the rubber ring in the wreckage that is my life.

I lift them. I hold them aloft. I breathe in. I place one foot in a leg. It slides. Then the second leg. So far, so good. I have a wire coat hanger on hand, just in case of emergencies. Ooh, here they go, over my knees. Over my thighs. Oh my God. Up and up they go, like a flag being hoisted up a greasy pole. Now over the arse. This is too easy! Are they the right pair? I swivel and twist, and I look at my arse in my skinny jeans and it looks … normal. Now, the moment of truth. I breathe out through my mouth as though practising to give birth again. Heh! Heh! Heh! My hands are sweating and so I wipe them on the denim. 'Come on. Don't let me down. You can do it.'

And I reach down, grasp the zip and pull it northwards. No flesh is trapped. There is no warping of little metal teeth. No grinding of my own. Finally, the button through the hole and – ta-dah! – I am in my skinny jeans.

Was it all worth it? The expense, the pain, the betrayal, the humiliation? For the simple pleasure of putting on a pair of trousers.

Well, yes. Sort of.

After Beardgate, I sat in my house, hands on my knees, telly off, waiting. I opened the Sonos app, played Sade's 'No Ordinary Love', but got too red around the gills and had to turn it off. There's nothing like. You and I. Baby.

There were signs, of course, and not just the lack of sex and the ironed tea towels. The carefully folded and colour-coordinated Smedley sweaters. The huge tranches of time spent in the bathroom. The fact he married me, when he is so handsome. The lack of sex – did I mention that? The silences. The disappearances. The resentment. The psychic friend of Neps's sister who'd once told me one of the men in my life is '70% gay'. The fact he admitted, and I've only just remembered this, that he had gone on holiday to Venice not long after we met and had snogged a man. I had dismissed it as just a blip or youthful experimentation, as he had said, 'But I didn't get an erection', as if that made it okay.

How duplicitous. That was a sign, surely. A Billboard Outside My Misery.

I sat and I sat. At one point, I got up and lifted my wedding photo from the mantelpiece: searching for clues, trying to make myself even more miserable, I suppose, winding up that little spring of stress even tighter. And then it hit me. Why his best friend Rishi had been so odd around me. Why he disappeared. Why he refused to be best man. I thought it was because he hated me, because of course I was hateful. But I realised his coldness, his sullenness around me, was because he knew Neps was gay. It was his best friend's dubious morals he disapproved of. Not my size. Not my race. And oh my God. The dried mud on the hem of his jeans. I've read Alan Hollinghurst, I'm not that stupid. The mud meant he had been cruising on Hampstead Heath.

I had thought he might phone, but there were no missed calls, nothing in my inbox. Just a text from the Kennington Tandoori. At least they love me. Finally, at about 10 p.m., just when I'd given up hope and decided to put my nightie on, I heard his key in the door. I could not wait to tell him his bags are packed and upstairs. I was still too sore to lug them down to the front door, my first choice.

'Hi,' he said, looking sheepish. I actually expected him to start bleating. He placed his keys on the table by the front door. 'Listen …'

I was artificially bright and brittle.

'Can you do me a favour? Fetch the holdall from upstairs?'

'Why, where are you going? Where are the babies?'

Tears were welling in his huge eyes, but I had to ignore this. I had to think of myself. My babies. Myself, mainly. Because if I'm not okay, they are not okay.

'I'm not going anywhere. You're the one who's leaving.'

I moved to stand in the hallway and I opened the front door. He backed out of my way, genuinely scared, and loped up the stairs. While he was rummaging around, probably locating his beard trimmer, I grabbed his wretched bicycle, the ruiner of so much knitwear, the scuffer of so many walls, the dripper of so many droplets of oil, and I propelled it out the door, down the steps and into the road, where it fell on its side, wheels spinning.

'Oi!' he said, emerging with a speed I'd not seen for a decade. 'Have you gone completely mad? What on earth are you doing?'

'No straight man does yoga. What sort of not-even-husband but friend are you that you ignore me? You refuse to lift your eyes to look at me. You have sex with me with your eyes closed and your Apple AirPods in. You didn't even NOTICE that you were smothering me with my own breasts during birthday sex! Me having cosmetic surgery was YOUR FAULT! You made me feel that I was the bad person, when I always tried so hard to make you happy. You were never honest with me. What were you doing, snogging that ginger man? I know without a shadow of a doubt that you are gay.'

He looked shocked.

'At least try to go pale,' I told him.

He hung his head. 'I'm so sorry,' he said. 'I don't know what you think you saw, but it was nothing. I left because I didn't want a scene. It wasn't the right place. She didn't deserve her night to be ruined. Anyway,' and he was emboldened now, believing his own fantasy, 'how do you know? Even I'm not sure, not completely. All this dieting and surgery stuff has been difficult for me too you know.'

Jesus H. Christ. The fact he wants a dick in his mouth is now my fault. Of course it is. I told him I was fed up trying to please him. That he never, ever tried to please me. That I am tired of trying to push him up a hill.

'I do try. I did. Maybe if we both tried a bit harder? I don't want to lose you, or the babies.'

I placed both hands on my hips, or in the approximate place where my hip bones should be. Where they will be, one day. I didn't bother saying that I tried so hard over the years, that I am exhausted. That he has wasted my life. That he has made me doubt myself, and my sexuality (not that I was ever into women; just that I questioned how I could be so incredibly unattractive to my husband), and my sanity. That I am fed up cheeping 'Neps!' 'Neps!' I refused to tell him that he made me hate myself, because I've been doing that for a very long time. But not anymore. Instead, not wanting to be the victim a moment longer, 'I gave you all the love I had. You took my love,' I said, channelling Sade. 'But you know what? I don't chase. I *re*-place.'

With that, he looked defeated. He gathered a coat off the peg, shrugged it on. I think he was tired of lying, too.

'I still want to be in your life, see the twins.'

'Yes. Of course. I would never stop them from being with you. I know what being without a dad would do to them. Did to me.'

'I do love you, you know, Stick,' he said, his voice thick.

At this, I lost my cool. Because I know it's not true. If he had loved me, really loved me rather than just tolerated me, circumnavigated me, he would never have married me. He knew he was gay on my wedding day. And the awful thing is, if truth be told, I knew he was, too. I just didn't feel I was worthy of anything better.

'I want you to LEAVE!' I shouted at him, so loud the cat bolted, tail a toilet brush out the cat flap, breaking it in his haste.

And with that he was gone.

. . .

I took him back. Of course I did. Within less than 24 hours.

After that awful night of the long lies, he had the grace to leave without further fuss to give me the chance to calm down. I went upstairs to peer out the window at his retreating back on his (slightly bent, I have to be honest) bicycle. It turns out he went to stay with his lesbian friend in Barking (and, yes, she is indeed a dog), to give me some space and not disrupt the kids, who I told him were due home at any minute and would sniff out an argument as surely as an illicit bag of crisps.

But the next day, he called out of the blue. 'Baby, I love you so much,' he had sobbed down the phone.

And to my un-Cosmopolitan, un-woke, MeNeither shame, I had caved. Faced with the stark reality of being alone, I was terrified of the future, of having to cope with everything, even though deep down I knew he was a liability, a third child, a giant toddler. Fool that I am, and even my laptop is recoiling at this bit, I took him back. I even drove to pick him up. I think at the time I knew it was crazy, but a part of me didn't want the drama to end. It was like the interval in the Harry Potter play: instead of the audience thinking, 'Oh, goody, vodka and ice cream', we all just wail 'Noooo!'

So I collected him and his knitwear and trainers and laptop (I made sure we 'forgot' his bike in the lesbian's narrow hallway; let her cardis be snagged for the next six months, see how she puts up with it), we got back to the house and he walked around, as if seeing our home for the first time. He actually stroked the sofa and kissed the cat full on the nose. The twins came home from school, ran at him and hugged his legs, and he felt wanted. In a family. Safe. Normal. I think he realised how his life would be were he left to fend for himself in the LGBT dating pond, like a goldfish whose bowl has broken into a million pieces. His lesbian friend's house is typical of a left-wing mum who thinks it's beneath her to hoover: toys and cheap coats on the stairs, millions of crusty bottles in the bathroom that have never been used or dusted. Cat litter in the kitchen. Dead plants in the window box. I think he started to appreciate the hard work I put into making everything as nice and smooth for him as possible, like a slide in a playground. To him, I wasn't a wife, but one of those women in white who run backwards, levelling the ice for a game of curling. Whoosh! Whoosh! Here, have this and this and this. Don't bother your big head about that, let me deal with it. You sit down. Don't worry, I don't need an orgasm, let's make tonight all about YOU!

We made love that night he returned, too, me directing his mouth and hands to bits that were safe to land on. I wanted to prove a point. I wanted him to realise what he was letting go, what he had almost lost. He was even lovely to the twins, seeming to notice their big dark bulks for the first time. He told me he'd take them to a movie, give me a break. I almost cried with gratitude.

. . .

Things tick along. Life gets in the way. I let things slide. I oil his life again. Whoosh, off he goes in the playground that is a life constructed by women.

But of course, nothing is resolved. Is he still seeing Ginger Beard Man? Was that a blip? Is he straight now? Bi? Tri? What?

Problem is, I can't bring myself to ask him. I'm too scared.

Which is odd, really, as I am thinner than I've ever been, and I'd always imagined that once thin, things would automatically just slot into place, become easy: that I would be confident. The skinny jeans are now but a distant memory, destined for Oxfam to clothe the poor people who can't afford vegetables. I am now a size 14. If that were a text, that last line would be sent with fireworks. Weeeeee!!!

Problem is, the whole dieting thing is getting a little bit out of control. After the op, I was in so much pain I couldn't eat. I could merely suck pineapple juice through a paper straw. I then moved onto soup, just a little. And after a month, when it no longer hurt to chew or sit on the loo, I found I just didn't want food. It repulsed me. I would push along the smallest trolley in Sainsbury's and I couldn't bring myself to take things off shelves. It was as though I saw every bright little package for what it was: a drug. Evil. Maybe all that stuff is addictive and what'd happened is I had gone cold turkey.

Shocking, too, but I had somehow turned into one of those women who indulge in self-care, like Gwyneth Paltrow but with a smaller nose. My body was no longer a bin (a wheelie bin, if truth be told) into which I tipped all my sorrow, along with the twins' leftovers. It was now a temple: precious, fragile. One night, I actually had a dream where I was standing in the chapel at the St John and Elizabeth, doubled over with pain from the op, nauseous, and suddenly all the food I had ever eaten came back up, detritus in a river of lard: cheese and buttered naans; Walnut Whips and tubes of Pringles. Bread: hundreds and hundreds of loaves. Doughnuts. Orange Clubs. Penguins. Giant Buttons. Jaffa Cakes. I woke in a sweat. Why did I eat all that stuff? Why? I don't even like Jaffa Cakes.

It's all-consuming, this new body worship thing, though I'm consuming very little. I've even joined a gym and turned up for the yoga classes rather than just popping in to buy a sandwich. I still make sure I stand at the back of the class, too far away to see myself in the mirror. Not yet, not quite yet. I am not sure my creamy thighs quite stand up to scrutiny. But at least I only need one mat for my imprint. And last Saturday I even took the twins to swimming but, rather than stand in the gallery eating biscuits with the other mums, all of whom profess to be 'still losing the baby weight' even though their first one is now at university, I got changed into a black Speedo costume without demolishing the little changing room with my bulk. When I slipped into the water, I did not cause a tsunami. Whales and birds and elephants did not migrate inland, squawking and trumpeting. No one even turned to look at me. It was wonderful. To take part. To not have my children be ashamed of me.

It's such a novelty, you see, taking up so little space on the planet. Problem is, now I have a new body I sort of need somewhere exciting to take it. It's as if I've taken delivery of a Lamborghini and found myself stuck on the M25, during rush hour, in the rain, not sure which exit to take, when really I should be cruising the hills above the Amalfi coast, wind in my hair, a hunky, appreciative, tanned man by my side. A straight man.

Neps has noticed that I am diminished, of course he has. But I am not sure he approves. Being thinner (I am not thin, not yet) means I'm more mobile, which I don't think he likes. I am less apologetic, as I move lithely around the house, like a ballroom dancer.

And then an odd thing happened this morning at work. An email, from a name I didn't recognise, marked Confidential. Oooh.

I opened it.

'Hi! Hope you don't mind the direct missive. But I've been hearing lots of good things about you: the campaign to resurrect Topshop. And that event during Fashion Week, for bigger women on the catwalk? Inspired, and a great response on social media. I will cut to the chase. Ever since we met, briefly, at the F&F dinner at Petersham Nurseries, I've had you in mind for something. The fashion editor role, here at Marie Claire? Would that be something you would be interested in? I know you have super good contacts in Milan. Can we meet for a quick coffee and a chat?'

And so it is I am atop the OXO tower, with the silvery ribbon of the Thames as well as the world at my feet, discussing my 'package'. Oooh, err. Amazing, really. I am to have an assistant. An expense account. I am to go to all the shows with the editor.

At first, I'm reluctant, mainly because I'm scared. I tell her that my experience of styling and shooting fashion is limited. 'But look at you,' she said.

Oh God, what? Have I dribbled down my front? Has my period come early?

'You've put yourself, as a curvy girl, together really well. Am loving the slogan T, the flared jeans from a brand that uses less water than any other. You certainly know your stuff.'

I suppose I do. Since I turned 11 and discovered not just Vogue but Honey and 19 and Elle, I have studied fashion in a myopic way born of hankering desperately to look that way, one day. I'd become an expert at hiding my shape. I'd become an encyclopedia of which brands try and which brands are helmed by woman-haters. And now that I am smaller, I am simply enjoying the ease of getting dressed every day. The sheer fun of it. I think that's what she's finding good about me today.

But I'm still not convinced. What if one day all the lard returns? If I revert? Also, how will I manage the kids with so much travelling, especially now my marriage is unravelling? I am thinking all this in my head, but the publishing director, a tarty woman called Reenie with an over-baked cleavage and way too much jewellery, obviously reads my expression.

'It's a great big world out there,' she says.

And so I say yes to the job and yes to all the freebie dresses I will doubtless be getting. And freebie handbags. And town cars. And flowers left in my room. But still I am worried. About giving in my notice. About telling Neps. Why do even good things fill me with doubt?

When I get home, I'm not sure how to broach the subject. Most husbands – because he is still my husband, if in name only – would be thrilled, but … I'm not sure how he will take it. Me being away more. Having more money than him. Changing, while he remains the same.

But you know what? He's genuinely thrilled for me. 'You are so talented,' he says, opening a bottle of white, even though he's teetotal.

'But the travelling? New York, Milan, Paris, twice a year?' I haven't even told him about couture, cruise. Shoots in exotic locations.

'We'll cope,' he says.

And despite the cuckolding, I am thrilled he used the word 'we'. That he sees us as a team. It is only later, in bed wide awake and worrying at 3 a.m., do I realise the reason he'd seemed thrilled was the prospect of my prolonged absences.

. . .

I'm at Mum's, breaking the news. She looks worried.

'But can you leave him on his own?' she asks me, as though my husband isn't a man at all but a very chewy puppy. And this is a woman who has no idea he has cheated on me with anyone, let alone a man. (I haven't even told you this yet, too scared to do so in the age of MeToo, but when he came back after I chucked him out, I'd grilled him, like a rectangle of halloumi, and he finally admitted that he had 'done it both ways' with a man. And yet he is *still living in my house*.)

'But it's a great opportunity. More money. And the twins aren't babies anymore.'

'Yes,' she says, demonstrating that mums know everything. They have a sixth sense. A divining rod. 'But He's still a child.'

She tells me she's also worried I'm getting too thin. Honestly, you really can't please some people.

'Can't you stop now?' she asks me, worried tiny eyes boring into my soul. 'Your face looks a bit drawn.'

'No,' I tell her. 'I don't think I can.'

I leave, and only when I get into my car, search for my phone in my bag, do I realise she has secreted a packet of Rich Tea biscuits in there. I start to cry, now. How we push people away in our pursuit of perfection. How insulting, to reject her values, her nurturing, her stews. I'm sure she feels to blame. I make a mental note never, ever to tell her about Neps and Ginger Beard. It would break her. It would send her over the edge.

. . .

I take the job, of course I do. I'm not completely insane. My boss took the news quite well, told me, 'I always thought you were too creative to do PR.' The first few days in the office are a whirlwind. I've got two joint deputy fashion editors, one a redhead, one a brunette, who seem to job-share. Not something I'm overly happy with. An assistant called Karis, a tall, plain girl with spectacles who I soon learn wants to be a writer and is merely biding her time steaming clothes, attending 'appointments', putting Sellotape on the soles of shoes so they don't scuff and filling in my expenses claims.

The editor-in-chief of the magazine is another brittle blonde who bears the air of someone who knows she's not quite good enough and compensates for that by being overly self-promoting. Her editor's letters, all two pages of them, are full of, 'When I won my first award at the BSMEs [BSEs, more like: mad cows the lot of them!] last year …' and 'When I had tea with the Duchess of Sussex' and 'Why imposter syndrome is your own worst enemy: you deserve this', all the while professing the merits of mentoring while shafting the work experience girls by rewarding them with zero pay and learning the ropes of only how to fetch her zero-fat coffee.

But still. All is good. Neps is pulling his weight with the twins, and the household, the shopping and the cooking. It's amazing how much more men will do for you when you cease to expect anything from them.

We still occasionally have sex. It's odd, though, that despite me being a size 12 (sent with fireworks and confetti), I feel he's merely going through the motions. He still doesn't look at me too closely. I am just a warm body, a vessel to receive his fluids. Just as a child I had vacillated between Steve McQueen and Paul Newman in The Towering Inferno, agonising for weeks if not months over such a difficult choice of who I loved more and would want to ask me to marry them, now I veer between being absolutely certain that my husband loves me, it was just a blip, and waiting for him to grow a Freddie Mercury tache and start wearing tight white vests and heels.

I'm in Paris when the cashmere is pulled from my eyes. Oh God, I'm so ashamed.

Me and the team are staying at the Hotel Montalembert, almost opposite Diptyque. (I know. I'm sorry I've become so otherworldly. The people who work in fashion are so very good, you see, at turning heads, washing brains, which is the reason you keep visiting that sequinned jacket in Zara rather than doing any actual work. I actually went into Gucci the other day, spied a perfectly normal white shirt costing £350 and exclaimed, 'Wow, that's reasonable.' It's like a disease, honestly. A rather apt term, given the theme of this particular chapter, which you will find out shortly, so please don't fast-forward. Stay with me.)

The Montalembert is the very hotel Nancy Mitford's Fanny frequented in Don't Tell Alfred. The marble lobby still echoes with the sound of her tinkling laughter and acidic wit. Anyway, we'd just been to the Hermes show and then to an 'appointment' at the Dries store. How lovely, how novel (no one in fashion reads novels), not just to fit through the door, but to fit in the clothes!

We get back to the hotel and I suddenly have a burning sensation. I desperately need to go to the loo. The ancient lift is so slow in arriving, I abandon the girls and the packages and haul myself up the marble staircase to my room.

I barely get to the bathroom in time. The pain is off the wall. There is blood in the bowl. Oh no. I'm dying. All the surgery and the dieting and the sit-ups was for nothing. What on earth is happening?

I start Googling. Is it the honeymoon disease, you know, cystitis, the disease I didn't get when on my actual honeymoon? No. We haven't been doing it that much; twice, actually. Thrush? And, oh dear God, did the girls notice I rushed off? Did I leave a trail?

Will I be all over Twitter? 'Fashion editor floods lobby #shouldhaveboughtaTenalady #fannyflood.'

The next day, we take the Eurostar home and I feel fine, bar a slight pain in my nether regions and a general feeling of hotness. I wonder if one of my wounds has become infected. Did the surgeon leave a spanner inside? No. It's been too long. It can't be the surgery.

I get home. Neps is making dinner, the twins are in their room on their tablets which I was finally able to buy them and he pecks me on my forehead. 'Oh, you feel clammy,' he says.

'I'm fine.'

'Maybe you should get checked out? Maybe something got infected after all?'

I can't type this. I can't. I'm too ashamed.

And so, it is two days later that I emerge from the medical centre off Railton Road with a prescription and a terrible realisation of what exactly is going on in my life.

I have HPV. A sexually transmitted disease most commonly found 'in the gay community'. And as, unlike some people I could name in this book, I am not a Whore, it can only have come from one person. And that person is soon to be very homeless, and very familyless, and very alone, again. I realise I should have made him wear a condom or get checked out before I allowed him anywhere near me. But, and I am really sorry about this, there was a tiny little part of my brain that was thinking: 'I know. Another baby. Sod the surgery. That would do it. That would tie him to me. That would put a spanner in his works.'

It's my own damn, stupid, recidivist fault.

As I walk home, clutching my prescription (and my crotch, if truth be told; I still can't spend any length of time away from a bathroom) and my dignity, a Biggie Smalls song is playing loud from someone's open window. 'Baby give me one more chance.'

Not this time. Not this time.

CHAPTER TEN
The Pope's not even Italian!

Normally, the thought of getting dressed for work involves the sort of planning they went through for D-Day: enough stretchy black fabric to construct a hot air balloon; make sure my black opaque tights are washed and without not just actual ladders, but no bald bits where the pressure has proved too great. A ballet cardigan, the sort of unending hank of wool that has never and will never experience a pas de deux. I'm remembering how the fat me was so unpredictable, too: weight always seemed to have shifted in the night, like sandbanks, so I was never quite sure what would fit or what would explode, a cushion being used for rifle practice.

But now that I'm a size 12, there is no need for the boob weather map on a new day in Thin Land: I choose a bandeau black bra and black bikini pants from an impressive array of underwear, as insubstantial as leaves in autumn; my old underwear was pale pink and industrial, with corsets and gussets and steel rods of reinforcement; something you'd put on to restrain a lunatic in an asylum. Which is exactly what I was. Mad. To waste my twenties being fat.

It's funny, how the memory of what it is like to be me as a fat person is receding. The tugging of zips, the fist in the face when the zip, without warning, suddenly gives up the ghost, the laddering of tights, the wriggling, the pain in my ears as yet another too small garment is pulled over my head, the shoving of feet into flats, the disguising of the mono-boob with huge baubly necklaces, the throwing on of not so much pashminas as super-king-size throws. This morning, though, what with all the misery, the upset, the betrayal, the incontinence, everything just floats on, like that silk scarf in The Bodyguard. Everything seems to go with everything else. I could layer a cashmere tank under a mannish jacket (I can wear tailoring! And not look be mistaken for Jo Brand! Or Nicola Sturgeon! Or Ruth Davidson!) under a pea coat and still be as narrow as a blade of grass.

I'm now inside the Royal Opera House, Covent Garden. Even the journey had been a swift glide on a gondola through Venice: the admiring glances from men and women, small children and dogs. No one stood up on the bus to offer me their seat; instead, I could stand, for once not part of a subgroup that includes mums with pushchairs and people with no legs and arms or who are over 100 years old. Instead of barrelling along, head down, along the last bit of Oxford Street, I couldn't resist glancing sideways at my reflection in shop windows; at one point, I collided with a very handsome young man who had been looking down at his phone. But rather than swear at me, he actually licked his lips, and turned around to drink me in (given I'm now a shot of tequila, rather than a yard of ale).

There was a red carpet outside the Albert Hall, which I glided along as if on casters, turning this way and that for the photographers who shouted my name and begged for me to pose, teapot fashion. The one time, fat, I had braved a red carpet (for the premiere of The Aviator on Leicester Square; I'd been put in charge of shepherding Kate Beckinsale. The skinny bitch so got on my last nerves at the after-party, with public displays of affection for her latest beau, I was tempted to ask whether she intended to swallow him whole, python fashion), the photographers had all yelled at me, 'Get out of the way! Move your arse! You're blocking the light! You're causing a total eclipse of the sun!'

I spy one young man wearing a fur motorbike helmet, which he has yet to remove. The jostling for seats: I can't help but laugh when I notice one has the name 'Kate

Moose' on the back; I know fashion people are dim, but seriously. I settle myself in my allocated teeny gilt chair – they have misspelt my magazine as Marie Curie; yeah, we cure cancer as well as telling you 'the ten best things to buy for a small balcony!' – but I care little as I'm so thrilled my tiny arse doesn't even fill it; there is an actual margin. Normally – on a train, say – my arms would always overflow into the gangway; every few seconds, I would have to scrunch them in, and secure them to my sides, a free-range turkey trussed with strong string ready for the oven, to a chorus of indignant tuts and reallys and honestlys. Once, a woman was so enraged by the temerity of my arms taking up space in the aisle, she said, 'God only knows what you cost the NHS.' Fucking ugly bitch. She is probably so mean-spirited she's nursing cancer cells as we speak; we can but only hope. I know it's uncharitable, but she'd deserve it.

I notice with some alarm my seat is next to the one assigned to the editor of Vogue (or Vague, as some savant has written on the label on her seat). She is a sour-faced woman who always snubs conversation, preferring to read a memoir by someone she knows in her generous lap. But today, who knows, she might be open to a bit of banter or gossip. She might discover me, hire me, say, 'Hi, Pam! I've never noticed before, but you are now thin enough to get through the Revolving Door Challenge at Vogue House. Welcome on board!'

Oh dear God. Here she bloody well is.

She comes in to land in her seat, a Boeing 747 at Heathrow (she's not slight; I half expect little men in fluro jerkins and noise-cancelling ear protectors and great big paddles, guiding her down), imposes on my margins by about three dress sizes and surveys the scene grumpily around her. Who could possibly be grumpy, being the editor of Vague? Vogue? As she lobs her carrier bag of free hair products across the catwalk, striking a pink-haired blogger on the shoulder pads, a celebrity arrives. We know it is a celebrity, though we cannot see an actual person, as its essence is surrounded by a swarm of camera lights, and giant furry microphones, and downmarket women in kitten heels (the TV reporters) running backwards in front of it. I turn to my neighbour, as prickly as a porcupine. 'Have you any idea who that is?'

'What am I?' she snaps, planting enormous shades on her fat face. 'Human Google?'

I decide to leave it. Must be hard, toiling in that white office on Hanover Square every day, deciding which freebie to put on, wracking your brain for hours so you can eventually write on the cover: 'The new season, now!'

And then, out of the blue, she suddenly becomes all pally and says to me (or at least I think it's to me, unless she's boss-eyed as well as boring), 'I'm so late, I had to call them to postpone the first look [in fashion, clothes are never outfits or designs: they are 'looks']. Hyde Park was closed, due to the Pope's visit, if you please. And he's not even Italian!'

I murmur my sympathies. The lights dim and the miles of plastic covering the catwalk – there is to be a fashion show before the awards proper; oh, goody – is untaped and unfurled by minions (sod turtles and albatrosses; we in fashion deplore smudges) and the show begins, with music so loud all the tiny dogs in the front row are wearing huge ear protectors, like the ones worn by Gwyneth Paltrow's daughter, Apple, at Live 8. Models barely in their teens emerge from behind a huge white board, with the name of the designer of the year etched upon it in giant letters. They seem startled by the lights, the photographers, the crowd. You might think we in the front row are the elite, but only moments before, the photographers, all of whom are badly dressed and overweight and bald, dressed to a man and woman as though they are just off to fight the Taliban, had shouted at us to uncross our legs and 'move yer sodding 'andbags!' Seriously, you'd have thought we were nannies, or PRs. The models stalk down the catwalk, unsmiling, wobbling on their high shoes. You can see their nipples and their kidneys.

They pose at the end of the runway, this way, that way, challenging, pouting, presenting all the angles of a set square, before turning, desperate, almost, to disappear into the yawning mouth at the other end. Oh, how I had always wanted to be a model. I can see now even I'm not thin enough. I'm certainly no longer young enough. Jesus. Some of them are so recently out of the cradle I could swear they need nappies; a couple clearly need incubators. But what I love most though is their hair: so straight and blunt cut, so Calvin Klein, and shiny, like tempered chocolate. Once, when I was fat, I allowed some insane hair stylist to straighten my hair: people mistook me for Dawn French; even bus drivers shouted, 'Oi, where's Jen? How's Lenny?' I love, too, the models' huge eyes, making them resemble bush babies. Just gorgeous.

When the show is over, after barely five nanoseconds, the designer of the year emerges to take a bow and be pelted by calla lilies. I keep hoping one catches him at an odd angle, sending him into a coma. He is an obese, shaven-headed, short, tattooed gay man in a crumpled T-shirt, trainers and loose Levi's that reveal his arse cleavage. He obviously despises both women and fashion. He is preceded by a narrow line of models, a shepherd herding sheep not remotely fat enough to be transported live for halal slaughter. They are all applauding him, though God knows why. He is as short as a stump, while they are as tall as masts on a sailboat, as perfect as marigolds. He gives a perfunctory wave

165

and then disappears to hoover up more accolades and cocaine, probably.

It's interesting that while I once (what am I saying? Once. I should have typed 'always') thought eight and a half stone was what I wanted to be, after seeing the winner of model of the year, as frail as a sparrow after a particularly harsh winter, I am wondering, hmmm, perhaps I need to be under eight. She really is breathtaking, and rich. Millions of followers. I find I am so impressionable, as Thin Me, in a way Fat Me commendably never was; I now see a photo of Kate Moss at the Topshop Unique show in a pair of flared vintage jeans with a wide brown belt, hair the colour and texture of straw, and immediately I want to dash home, sling all the toothpick jeans out the window and mainline bleach.

As I leave, I bump into a fashion PR. I remember her for having once, when I was still fat but had managed to gate crash the Tom Ford show – the sort of event where they measure you with calipers at security to find out your BMI – told me, 'I'm sorry, we don't have enough room for you. Can you go over and stand by that wall?'

Today, though, given my increased status and decreased circumference, she mwah-mwahs me, then says, 'Wasn't the fashion moving? Oh, and by the way, really good news! You know my biggest client …'

I try to think. Do I? Um.

'You know, the client who pioneered organic, plant-based skin care, free from parabens? Who died of cancer? Well, it's his memorial at St Paul's next week. Would love it if you could come along.'

'Oh yes, great!' I reply. 'Sad, but great.'

. . .

As I push my way down the stairs through the crowds – the young men still wearing fur motorcycle helmets, the young women in fur, with pink hair, and Vuitton bumbags, and backless coats, and pyjamas as outerwear, and ironic leopard spot, all so desperate to be noticed, to be successful – I spy someone I recognise moving between the tables. It's the executive fashion editor of Marie Curie – goodness, even I'm calling it that now! I wonder if I am getting more stupid: does a low BMI equate with a low IQ?

Her role is to schmooze all the big, luxury brands and make sure we give them enough editorial coverage in exchange not just for advertising, but for allowing us to shoot their clothes. She has a chart in her office with every time a brand is mentioned, shot as a cut-out, given a full page or graced with the kudos of a cover noted on a graph. If ever a label is seen to dip in our level of coverage, she will berate the fashion team and tell us to up the ante.

And I had thought the pages were filled with good taste, not just good business. The big brands will even complain if they feel a celebrity shot in their designs is not deemed A-list. Or A-list and too old. Or A-list and too fat.

I'd always held this woman in awe as Fat Pam, to be honest. She was the only person in fashion and beauty who ever acknowledged my existence as a lowly PR; it was as though we were members of some very exclusive club: her, very old and grey; me, very overweight and pink. Hmm. Pink and grey do go well together. She knows everyone. She has been in the business for, what, 30 years? And yet here she is, moving from table to table, necking the dregs left in every champagne flute. She has no idea that I, her new (sort of) boss, is watching her and so I sneak out a side door to save her the embarrassment. But it's a sad, desperate moment. She has given her life to fashion, loved it, but it has never loved her back. She knows she is past it. She knows everyone thinks she is a joke. And as I exit into the crisp air of Covent Garden, I feel a chill, as though a ghost has just passed by me. I realise that could be me one day. In the blink of an eye. Shallow. Sozzled. Sad. Single. As I walk down towards Long Acre, I encounter a phalanx of paparazzi. For a second, I think they want to take my photo, so I pose, arms making the shape of a teapot. Then they shout, 'Get out the way! Pixie! Pixie!' I am fashion roadkill. Gosh, that feeling of fitting in didn't last long, did it?

8¹/₂ STONE

CHAPTER 11
Oh. My. God. I look like Gollum!

After I got the STD diagnosis and threw Neps out, he didn't even come back for the rest of his things. He didn't even desert me properly. He left behind some really annoying things, like a cat spraying a bush with urine: the complete works of Keats. A book on the Enlightenment. A really horrible inflatable chair. Paper clips. Skin cells.

Why does every single aspect of a relationship – courtship (flirting, texting, enthusiasm, sexiness, life-story telling, willingness, waxedness, hair dyeing, teeth cleaning, lawn returfing, clothes buying, listening to their awful, boring anecdotes with an interested expression, head on one side, sucking and not gagging, moaning, laughing), wedding (hen weekending, ring buying, Smythsons visiting, calligrapher hiring, licking and stamping and posting, flower meeting, menu choosing, dieting, dress fitting, cake recipe approving, placement placing, hours spent poring over glass cases at a snotty jeweller's on Old Bond Street, music booking, readings assigning, speech writing, flower disposing), honeymoon (flight booking and paying for, seat choosing, parking, making a note of exactly where we bloody well parked, car hiring, finca borrowing from friend who will doubtless want payment in some form, map drawing, money changing, waxing, swimwear buying, navigating, fishing the deceased lizard out of the pool) and even now splitting up – fall to me!

Why, when Neps cheated on me WITH A MAN, BOTH WAYS, REMEMBER, WITHOUT WEARING A CONDOM, did I have to hire a divorce lawyer, when he is the one who is the serial cheater, the liar? My God, when I went to meet her ¬– a lovely woman called Emma who annoyed me slightly by only working three days a week – she even said there is a possibility I would have to pay him alimony as I now earn so much more than he does (not difficult), and that he would be entitled to half my home! When he has never, ever paid the mortgage! Or the council tax. Or utilities. Or the window cleaner. Or the parking permit. Or the boiler insurance. Or furniture. Or Sainsbury's. Or the nappy and Sudocrem bill in Boots. In one of our protracted discussions post wee-gate, mainly conducted in my solicitor's office, he admitted a man had been in our bed on the night I went under the knife (he had deposited the twins with my mum) as, and I quote, 'I had felt betrayed, and horribly abandoned.' I can only hope he broke the habit of a lifetime and changed the sheets. Oh, yes, he did, didn't he? So, that is why the lamp was wonky: vigorous sex. The earth moved. As did the furniture.

How can that be fair! God, if I'd murdered someone I swear I'd be treated better. And be in prison. At least then I wouldn't have to whizz round Lidl and defrost the freezer.

Anyway. Sod him. I'm not in love. Don't you forget it. And so, needing a bit of space and time to think, I accept an invitation from the PR for Tod's to spend a long weekend in Capri. Did you know the correct way to pronounce it is with the emphasis on the 'Cap', not the 'ri'? No, neither did I. But now that I am a size 12 and falling, I know these things. I have gained entry to a Whole New World.

I arrive at Stansted with my vintage Vuitton tote, relieved to be away from everyone. This is the first holiday I have taken thin. I've been so excited I even went shopping for a whole new outfit. Shops! A world of possibilities, rather than being what they had been up till now: an assault course. The Battle of the Bulge. A place (Evans, usually) where I would crawl, on my three bellies, pulling myself by my elbows through mud to find something, anything that would go on past my head. Where I would be hit by the shrapnel – rat-a-tat-a-tat – of the sharp, barbed looks from the shop assistant. 'It's all right for you,' I thought but didn't say when a burqa-clad assistant in Zara warned me not to rip anything or burst any buttons or leak on any gussets because I would still have to pay for it. 'You could be Two Ton Tessie and no one would be any the wiser.' Maybe I should have not opted for surgery but simply moved to Kabul instead.

A small group of 'journalists' are huddled by the check-in, while a young PR takes everyone's passports. I always wonder on these jaunts how quickly adult women become infantilised, totally dependent on the child who is now to look after them.

'Hi!' I say brightly, putting down my bag, shoving my The Row sunnies back in my expensively highlighted hair. I know I look good. I know they all know who I am. I know the PR is a little bit scared. 'I'm Pam. From Marie Curie.'

Oh dear. I must stop saying that. 'Hi!' everyone says. I notice there is a man in the group. A thin white duke of a person, in combat gear. He is looking at his feet. I wonder if he's a photographer, the only straight men who are not extinct in the privileged pool I now swim in.

'And you are?' I say, extending a French-manicured hand. A thin gold bracelet round my wrist that says one word: 'Success.'

'I'm Jeremy. I loved the joke, by the way.'

'Which one?' I have so many.

'The one about curing cancer.'

Hmmm. Could I have just met someone who finally gets me?

. . .

The hotel is gorgeous. We landed last night, exhausted, and were ferried to a place near the coast, where we'd stay for just one night. A giant moon hung heavy in the sky, huge and orange, reminding me just a little of a pizza. It is Naples, after all. Early the next morning, we all got on board the ferry that would take us to the island of CAPri. I sat on deck, wind in my hair, not caring about anything for once. Just caught up in the beauty of everything.

At the dock, we disembarked into quaint little old taxis with stripy canopies and we wound up and up, higher and higher, until we got to the Palace hotel. I noticed I was in the cab containing Jeremy. I think he might just have engineered that. I could feel his breath on the back of my neck, like a little fan. Maybe he is a fan. Of me.

'Now,' the baby PR had said, 'one of you is lucky enough to have the room with the private pool and it is … Jeremy!'

He had the decency to blush.

We spent the day by the pool and now, as evening falls, we are in two stripy taxis, on our way to dinner. I've chosen my outfit carefully: a nude body-con and a pair of Louboutin heels that are as narrow as my torso, the red tongue of the sole poised to tell everyone in the world behind my retreating back that I have much more money than sense.

There is only one spanner in the works. As I was getting dressed earlier, I accidentally caught sight of myself in the full-length mirror in my room. This is the problem with hotels, you see: they never give you enough time to make friends with the mirror. The bellboy always shows you the minibar, the balcony and how to use the TV, but he never, ever throws a scarf over the full-length mirror, warning, 'This little bastard will age you by a century.' (Oh God. Ageing. Is that all I have to look forward to? I will just get over adult acne and be pitched into wrinkles, blindness and a whiskery chin.)

As I saw myself in the mirror, it was as though a stranger had suddenly gained entry with a duplicate key. I didn't recognise what I saw. 'Oh. My. God.' I exclaimed, taking it all in, my hand shooting to my mouth. 'I look like Gollum!'

I've gone too far, surely. There I was imagining I'm Karlie Kloss, but in reality, I'm like cauliflower couscous: all white and knobbly.

I pulled on a Herve Leger bandage dress. Oh, the irony that it is called a bandage dress, because if you could fit inside this little baby you would never, ever be in need of surgery. I gingerly surveyed my form in the mirror, being careful to cut off my head, as I'm still not sure my head is having the desired effect: it's still pink and a little bit round. But I have to say, the rest is good when I've got clothes on. I'm Vanessa Paradis, nonchalant and soignée, swaying and singing Joe Le Taxi on Top of the Pops. If only I were French and had a gap between my two front teeth. If only I were still in my twenties. No, no. Stop. Stop. This is enough. This is better.

As we draw nearer to the Locanda the road is lit by candles, hundreds of them, flickering our way. I'm sure they can't be good for air quality or global warming or forest wildfires, but still. It's a lovely touch. We are now seated at big tables, beneath huge trees heavily pregnant with oranges and lemons. I'm next to Jeremy. I swear that at one point his brown, hairy knee (he is wearing combat shorts) touches my leg. I know I slightly resemble a collapsed umbrella. All edges. I am someone Bob Geldof would be very concerned about. But I suddenly feel as lithe and gravity-defying as Olga Korbut; I'm tempted to tie up my hair in jaunty pigtails and perform a backwards flip from the parallel bars.

We are given thimbles of limoncello. I sip mine, but I notice he downs his in one. Then another. Perhaps he's nervous. I find out he's a travel writer, though what he really wants to do is write a novel.

'What would it be about?' I ask him.

'Oh. Sex. Relationships. Disappointment. Betrayal.'

'Oh, a romcom.' And he laughs.

We finally head back to the hotel. I'd only picked at my pasta, which is a change, really, when once I'd have inhaled it. I'm in the back with Jeremy and someone from Hello! (I really wish they'd say, Goodbye!) The young PR is wittering away in the front.

'So!' she says to me. 'Are you married? Any kids?'

I don't want to say, but I suppose I have to, given Google's been invented, the annoying Californian bastards. How, I often wonder, will anyone ever be able to lie again? 'Um. Yes. Two. They are quite small.' I don't want him thinking my vagina is the size of China. 'And I am getting divorced. In fact, it's almost finalised.'

'So, you are a bit battered and bruised,' he says. I can no longer see his face as it's quite dark, which somehow makes me braver, as though he doesn't really exist.

'Hope to be later,' I say foxily; I have no idea where that came from. That limoncello must be stronger than I thought. I must be getting drunk because I have fewer square inches to soak it all up. I can feel him shifting in his seat. I swear his trousers move.

Everyone snakes into the bar, which is lovely, and marble. My skin is still tingling from the day's sun.

'What would you like?' Jeremy asks me.

'No more limoncello, it's so strong!' I tell him. 'Just champagne. Please.'

While he waits for the drinks, he gets out a packet of cigarettes, lights up. Now, if Neps had ever done that, I'd have rugby tackled him, berated him, accused him of wanting to burn my babies in their beds. But I don't know, tonight I don't care. I find his smoking attractive. Sexy. Dangerous.

We sit in a corner and chat. Which is how he ends up asking me up to his room to 'try out my pool'. I feel like diving into his eyes: blue and small, slightly pig-like: the exact opposite of my husband's.

'My bikini is in my room, it's not dry,' I tell him.

'You won't need it,' he says.

And so I follow him. It's all very natural. He even reaches a skinny brown hand behind him that I'm meant to grasp, like an elephant. We get to his door. He places his key card at the entrance. 'Ooh, I have a green light,' he says saucily. I like his humour. Unlike Neps, he doesn't seem to have the weight of the world on his shoulders.

We go into his room. It's the usual mess that men make: clothes everywhere, sandals, towels, coins. But for a change I don't care. I don't care about anything.

'Look. Come see.'

He opens some curtains and double doors to reveal a small pool. The water is lit from below and is turquoise. I lean down, place a few fingers in the water. It is warm. Inviting. I really hope I'm not so drunk I throw up and get sick in my hair.

'Let me get you a drink,' he says, and he returns with a bottle.

I sit on the side of the pool, my feet now in the water. I secure my hair in a high ponytail, exposing my cheekbones. Who knew, really, that beneath all of that flesh I was in possession of an actual skeleton? I had assumed I was solid: a rolled and boned ham.

He sits down next to me.

'Take your dress off,' he says.

I can't. I really can't. I am okay in clothes, normal. But without them, he will see the scars, he won't be able to miss them. He will meet Gollum. My breasts are still too big. Smaller than they were, what with all the stress and the upset and the cuckolding, not to mention the Pilates, but when not restrained in a bra they can still go a bit free-range. Plus, I have some silver stretch marks on my thighs that will never go away – and believe me, I've tried. I'm waxed, but it's been seven days, so I am sure a few little bastards are emerging from their pores, like asparagus.

I don't say any of this. I just look, well, frigid. Frightened.

Thing is, he takes absolutely no notice. He starts to undo me, in more ways than one. He gently lifts my dress from me, discards it. I am now in bra and knickers. I wish I could reach the great big cushion, over there, and hold it over my tummy, like a shield.

'You are so beautiful,' he says, stroking my skin. He runs one hand down my arm.

'I'm not,' I say.

And then he kisses me. I dare to peek at him, and his eyes are closed. But as our lips part, he opens them, drinks me in. He undoes my bra and starts to suck on my nipples. It hurts, but I suppress the 'Ow!' I look down at him and realise we don't look like a cow with her suckling calf, but like a man and a woman. There is no resentment about him, no obligation.

'Let's get in the water!' he says, and with relief I slip into the small, square pool of blue light: no longer a walrus, today just a seal. He splashes in beside me and I realise he must be quite drunk. 'Oh, blimey!' he says, sinking suddenly. 'I'm still in my combats! All the pockets are filling with water! Help! Gahhh!'

And so, I do. I help him out of them. And just like that, we fall in love. It's like that scene between Woody Allen and Diane Keaton in Manhattan, where they are sat on a bench by the 59th Street Bridge watching the dawn come up. We sit by the pool, him in a robe, me in one of his sweaters, and I feel like a movie star. That's better than feeling like the Pillsbury Doughboy, surely? Isn't it?

. . .

It was so strange, having sex for the first time as a thin person. No need for it all to be done in the dark, like badgers. Whenever it looked like Neps was feeling frisky, I'd been known to unscrew light bulbs. Oh, for a three-day week! Bring back Ted Heath is what I say! The way Jeremy opened up my body, like the old me would lift the lid on a pizza box: full of wonder, anticipation, admiration, but with a bit less sniffing and chewing. Okay, a little bit of chewing. I am his ultra-thin and crispy base.

Once out of the pool he had led me over to the bed. He moved me higher up the pillows and it was so easy! There was no grunting with effort, from him or from me. No cranes. No hiring of forklift trucks. Often, when I was big, Neps would go to move me and then would just give up, thwarted, like someone delivering plate glass windows on Grand Designs, and say, 'Why don't you just stay where you are. I'll work around you.'

I am now a small blonde dot. The centre of this

new man's universe. I am no longer a planet with an equator. I am a new moon. I am a sliver. I am desirable. I am enough. Oh. My. God. Irene Cara, you were so completely right all along. What a feeling.

It was light enough for me to watch his face while he was making love to me and I was amazed to see he was smiling to himself. He was just so happy to be there. Neps always looked grizzly, like a baby with a full nappy. As if he were doing me a favour. And you know what? Here is the delightful thing. Jeremy didn't ask about my scars, or dash off to his laptop to Google them; he just ran a cool digit the length of them and then he kissed them. I even angled my rump at him so he could see the pale rivers of stretch marks, the orange-peel skin that no amount of dieting will ever eradicate, and for a moment he looked up at me and said, 'I love that you lived. You loved. You were hurt. But you survived.'

What a revelation. Being in bed with a man and I am not pulling the duvet over me, worried about wobbly bits, my stomach the colour and texture of Wensleydale cheese and probably full of it, too. The mattress no longer tilted. I was wearing a thong – before, that is, he took it off, which was so easy as, miraculously, it hadn't become a sheep in a bog. I wondered, briefly, a thought almost as brief as my knickers, whether the reason men fancy thin women is because we are more like boys, less like cows with udders. Less like their mums. I pushed the thought aside. No. I wanted this. I wanted this body. Just enjoy it. Inhabit it. Learn to live in the moment.

. . .

The next day, as we stood waiting for the jaunty taxi to take us back to the bay and the boat, all the others knew that we'd been at it. They could just tell. His grin was as wide as my old arse. I was embarrassed, plus my face was scarlet from his stubble, though I tried to blame it on the sun.

On the plane, in the clouds, I had that feeling I always get: I'm free of all my problems. That all my problems are down there. On earth. Far, far away. Where they can't possibly hurt me.

When we landed, of course, reality came crashing in like that bloody flood water. We shared a cab back to London and he kept holding my hand.

'But you are single, yes?'

'Well, yes.'

'And he's moved out, you know, to be with the other woman?'

I haven't yet told him my husband cheated on me with another man. It seems too sordid, too much. Like telling him I'm such an unlovable freak, I actually turned my husband to The Other Side.

'Yeah. I don't know. He's still around a lot, as the

house is near his school; I'm not a paedophile, he's a teacher. The twins love him, so I don't want to rock the boat too much. And the divorce is proving tricky. Did you know that divorces are now no-fault, that no matter he cheated on me, I might have to pay him alimony?'

The colour drains from his face. He is just so sweet.

'No!'

'Yes!'

. . .

It's now three months later. I've been spending as much time with Jeremy as my job and the twins and looking after my mum will allow. Neps knows I'm seeing someone, but he hasn't said a word. He is being really good with helping. Shopping, school run. He has even discovered how to start the lawnmower. I caught him Googling the instructions one day. 'Who knew you had to press the little blister to encourage the fuel?' he said, fascinated. Maybe this is what works with men. When we are in love with them, we expect too much. When we no longer expect anything from them, they surprise us.

'So why don't you move in with me?'

Jeremy has just asked me this. We are in his flat. It's lovely. Bare and minimal and impossibly urban. But lovely. No child detritus.

I tell him I can't. That it's too far from the kids' school. That, well … I couldn't think of another reason. 'Oh, you don't have a garden!' I say.

And he replies, 'What are they? Labradors?'

'Why don't you reverse things?' he says, propping himself on his elbows, so happy with himself that he has just had a terrific idea. I just love all the angles of him. His floppy hair. His straight nose. I love that he doesn't make me feel bad about myself. That there is no racial tension between us. It was so odd, seeing a white man's penis for the first time. My husband's is thick, and short, and stubby, emerging from an impenetrable forest of wiry black hair. While Jeremy's is long and elegant, with barely any hair at all. There is hardly any hair on him, if truth be told: a fuzz on his chest. A sheen on his arms. Nothing on his thighs. He is slightly girlish, though I would never tell him that. But rather than put me off, it just means I've become more open with him than I ever was with Neps, who with his huge brain if not huge dick always meant I was careful around him. Jeremy is just more straightforward. Old-fashioned. He opens car doors for me. He brings me cups of tea. He looks at me with love in his eyes, not resentment. He has never, ever brought me a long-dead spider. I always felt, with Neps, a bit like a jailer. All I needed was a huge set of keys.

It was Neps's difference that made me fall in love with him, at first, that afternoon after yoga when he'd asked me for coffee. But thinking hard now, rummaging around in my brain, I think I chose him because I believed no white man would have me. It's a terrible thing to say, but I married him because some tiny little hundred-years-old part of me felt he might think me worthy of him because I am white. God, how wrong could I have been.

'Reverse things how?'

'Well, usually the dad gets the weekends. Why doesn't he have them in the week and you get the weekends? The fun part. When you aren't at work and you're with me!'

And so that's how we did it. I moved in with Jeremy, taking enough of the twins' things for weekends: his office became their bedroom. He was welcoming, helpful. He made space in his wardrobe for my work attire (I left all the old too big sails and tents and marquees in Brixton), told me his Wi-Fi code, emptied a shelf in the bathroom for my unguents. But when two narrow beds were delivered for the twins and were placed in his office and he found he had to turn sideways to get to his desk, I swear his face clouded over and set slightly, as if I had, as old, fat me, just made a meringue and taken it past the point of soft peaks and into the dry and the chalky. Not nice at all.

And Neps got the house during the week. My only stipulation was that he was not allowed to invite his boyfriend to stay until after I'd picked them up on a Friday night. He agreed. He was happy. I was happy.

With my minimal new life. My working day was transformed: I could shift down a gear. I am now one of the winners in life, surely. The only thing I ever won as a child was 'Best-dressed wooden spoon' at the horticultural summer show and even then I cheated, dressing my spoon in my Sindy doll's equestrian outfit (fawn jodhpurs, checked shirt, tweed jacket, velvet cap) complete with one little rubber riding boot shoved on the handle.

What, really, now I'm thin and desirable and sorted and successful, could possibly go wrong?

CHAPTER 12
Where's the baby? Where is it?

It's Jeremy's birthday. And I have arranged a surprise!

On a hot Thursday morning, we get into my car. I've taken the day off. He doesn't have any freelance pieces to write. Oh, did I not tell you this bit? Are you sure I didn't? That I've agreed he can scale back on the freelance work, which will mean him travelling less, in order to write his novel? I will contribute more to his flat: groceries, utilities. I'm sure I told you that. Did I not? Anyway. It's all good. It really is, I promise you.

He's driving. I've packed the following: a Victoria Beckham black strappy dress with an asymmetric hem (borrowed – although in fashion parlance, we say we have 'called in' an item, never borrowed or nicked it). A bikini by She Made Me; it's crocheted which means I doubt I should get it wet. Heels. To travel I'm wearing inky flares and a sheer blouse by Valentino. I'm looking gooood. It is just one night, which is all I can afford, but I've made sure it will be special: champagne in the room, dinner at 8.30 p.m. Lunch the next day in the greenhouse.

I read out the satnav code. He types it in. Slowly. Carefully. With one forefinger. Why is everything men do done slowly?

'Oh, it's Lime Wood,' he says. 'In the New Forest.'

'How in God's name do you know that?' I say, aghast.

'I've been there before. On a freebie. Travel piece for GQ. They gave me the best room, the one with the bath at the end of the bed. But it's lovely. It will be great!'

Oh dear. I wasn't able to get that room. Fully booked. And strange, that he would have been dispatched to Lime Wood by a men's magazine, alone, when it's meant for couples. And Jeremy usually does the sort of travel writing that is like war reporting but without the danger: boot camp in the Mojave desert. Rehab in Rio. You know, macho holiday pieces in the Hemingway school, rather than the sort of feminine stuff I'm party to. The only reason he was in CAPri, it turned out, was because his editor wanted him to 'drink his way across Italy'. Must be hard, being a man, when everyone wants you to be Steve McQueen. At least when women are admonished to be more like Kendall Jenner they don't have to learn to ride a vintage motorbike. But the room I have managed to get is lovely, too: in the main house, not in an annexe.

. . .

We'd spent last weekend in 'early celebrations' at his parents' house in East Sussex: a thirties mansion, with all the usual rich people's accessories: a circular drive. Electric gates. A drinks trolley. Proper paintings, not just a reproduction of The Hay Wain. They even had little croquet hoops on the lawn. I wonder if people realise that they are clichés, with no taste of their own.

I'm always envious, though, of the way his family is with each other (I say 'always', but this was the first time I'd been graced with an invite). They stand around a huge island in the kitchen, heads thrown back, laughing, drinking cocktails made with obscure brands of gin, with things like home-grown mint and juniper berries lobbed in, some banquet or other slung in the pistachio Aga, dogs on cushions, everyone batting loud opinions on politics to one another; when all Mum and I ever did on special occasions was balance a tray on our knees (those awful, padded trays, with a painting of kittens playing with wool balls on the front), watching Long Lost Family on ITV, or Pointless, our only conversations about how much we like Alexander Armstrong while the other one's too tall.

His sisters, one still at school, one at uni, are blonde and tall and confident. I ask the little one what she's studying. 'Oh, fashion, fine art, politics. I might be a political correspondent on TV, that could be good, though I wouldn't put up with the trolling. I might want to work in fashion one day, too, but, you know, I'm not sure. It's all so irrelevant these days, doncha think? I get everything I own from charity shops. Far more sustainable.'

Okay. Thanks for that.

I'd been so looking forward to impressing his family. I'd arrived in pressed inky jeans, a 'called in' Barbour over a Peter Pan collar and hiking boots. Only when we were greeted at the door (huge, a porch stuffed with dirty wellies and umbrellas and old coats) did I realise I resembled none other than Kate Middleton, when everyone else was Kate Moss at Glastonbury, all oversized Viyella men's shirts with long-darned holes and floppy tea dresses over hobnail boots. These people have not a care in the world. They are warm and welcoming and chatty, not stiff at all. His dad is an older version of Jeremy: all sinewy and tall. His mum is blonde and brash. They actually have a housekeeper, who hovered (and hoovered) in the background. I felt less bad, then, what with the wafting smell of dead animal coming from the Aga, about nudging Jeremy, asking him to please remind his mum I'm vegetarian.

Annoyance crossed his lovely face. Two vats of some exotic gin in, he was tiddly, and I realised he was showing off to his family. Trouble is, I wasn't quite the prize they were expecting: more of a marrow than a rose, had this been the local horticultural show. I thought, with guilt, of how glad I was I hadn't brought the twins: it would have been like lobbing Rebel Wilson and Matt Lucas onto the set of Love Island. Neps of course was thrilled to get extra time with them, and anyway had been worried that exposing them to an upper-middle-class environment would make them want to join the Brownies, an organisation he of course believes is racist. They would doubtless be too big for the chairs, the narrow stairs up to 'the party floor'. What with all the skiing and horse riding and striding and talking, I doubt anyone in Jeremy's family tree has a BMI above that of a radish. I think I did 12k without even leaving the house.

Dinner was deafening. No one offered to put the TV on, which was probably black and white with an indoor aerial anyway. As the evening wore on, I started to wonder what Jeremy saw in me. He could have had some red-faced gal with a Labrador and acres. When we at last climbed up to bed, I noticed he stumbled, and as he'd brought his gin, it sloshed up the wall. 'Careful! You're spilling it!' I hissed.

'Oh, who cares.'

We had our own bathroom across the hall. I showered and put on my nightie. There was so much of everything: towels. Unguents. No wonder he's so careless. My mum would always render the last bits

193

of the Imperial Leather stuck to the label, moulding them into something useable.

He was on top of the duvet, naked, when I emerged. He patted the bed next to him naughtily. The thought of having sex with his family so near was something I hadn't even countenanced. So, I'd said, making a little joke, 'We can't desiccate your old room!'

But he'd missed it, and had rolled his eyes. 'Dear God. Did you ever go to uni at all?'

He knows I've merely been to fashion college. Why bring that up now? He was doubtless tutored, shoehorned into his place reading English. I wonder with all that education he hadn't learned that kindness is a virtue.

. . .

We drive west along the M4, then M25, M3. It's hot. He opens the sunroof, lights up a fag.

After almost three hours, we arrive at the hotel. 'Look!' I say, suddenly 12 again. 'Ponies!'

We leave the car by the entrance and check in. The lobby has a large circular table in the centre, upon which is balanced a flower display the size of a hippo, and a roaring open fire. Despite the fact it is me who has just handed the young woman my card, she goes to give him a piece of paper to sign. Fucking patriarchal society. He cocks his head towards me in a gesture I feel for some can't-quite-put-my-finger-on-it reason is slightly obscene. I feel like saying, 'Who am I? The cat's mother?' We are shown to our room, and when he walks into the marble bathroom, he has the grace to say, 'Wow!'

Left alone, we change into our swimwear, for all the world like Miss World contestants. At the pool area in the spa, reclined by the hot tub, we order drinks. A mojito for him, champagne for me; I figure champagne has fewer calories than anything else bar water, of course. Or nothing.

He says he's peckish, so asks the waitress if we can have some snacks. 'I'm afraid it's a food-free zone,' she says, and to my shock he replies, gesturing at me with a cocked thumb, 'A bit like her.'

I'm the cat's mother again! Give me a bowl of milk, why don't you? A collar with a bell! I know he finds my extreme carefulness around food … annoying. But I don't think he understands what it is to be a bigger woman in the modern world. How I cannot go back there. And I also know that were I to put the weight back on, he would leave me in a nanosecond. For the moment, I am a status symbol. Useful. Convenient, like long-life milk. But I know he would prefer for that symbol to be effortless. Just like all men want us to look as if we have just emerged from the shower, slung on jeans and a T-shirt, and still be beautiful. If they were to find out about the hair dyeing, the waxing, the primer, the concealer, the fake tan, the acrylic nails, the laser hair removal, the pore strip on the nose, it would all collapse, like a house of cards. Or my old arse.

Up in the room just now, changing, unpacking, he had hugged me then said something odd. 'You know what I find most attractive in a woman? Someone who can live in the moment. Not worry about tomorrow.'

Which of course as we all know isn't me at all. Which is why I am trying not to look at my phone. It's not that I'm worried about work, it is just that when you are a mum, you are supposed to check your phone every five seconds. It's the law. If you don't do that, Apple sends a report direct to social services and you are arrested. Because anything might have happened to them. A kidnapping, literally. Meningitis. A traffic accident. Why on earth is he being a baby, about my babies?

So, instead, my phone is in my bag, up in the lovely £545-a-night room not including dinner or breakfast. He orders another mojito. I try to relax. I pass the time looking at all the other women, reclining on sunloungers, reading, swimming, napping. Not one has a perfect body. Some are overweight, one looks pregnant. There are varicose veins. Grey hair. Really awful flip-flops. Saggy arms. But each and every one has a man by her side. An adoring man. A solicitous man. One couple are even playing cards. Each and every woman walks around, not a care in the world, no shame, no sarong and, as Mary J Blige would say, no drama. Completely comfortable in their near-nakedness. Like day-old babies.

We return to our room as the sun fades. By the pool, I had put on my trackie bottoms while still sitting down. Wriggle, wriggle, wriggle. Tug, tug, tug. A reverse, inept striptease. Old habits die hard. 'For heaven's sake,' he had said. 'What on earth is wrong with you?'

He opens the champagne I'd requested for his birthday, pours me a glass, spilling a little, but then makes himself a G&T from the minibar, which will of course cost me extra. But I say nothing. In the immortal words of Bros, nothing at all.

He manoeuvres me onto the bed. He has uttered barely a word. A tiny, tenacious weed grows in my brain: why, whether fat or thin, am I with men who are as monosyllabic and private as a potato? Why do I have to tiptoe round them, as though they are volatile, and I am Princess Diana, walking in chinos and a visor through a minefield? Why does no one tiptoe around me?

'C'mon,' he says now, shaking the water from his hair, positioning me, moving limbs, strands of hair, as though I'm a supermodel on a photo shoot. But it all feels as though he is doing it because he feels obliged to, as it's his birthday in a posh hotel and he has to humour me, play a part, play along. He points the bedside lamp at me, lifts up my tiny T-shirt, mimes peering down a telescope; his little joke about my breasts having shrunk a bit. 'Are you ready for your close-up? Let me see that gorgeous body. You remind me of Sigourney Weaver, in those little pants and T-shirt. So lithe and fearless. You BIIIITCH!'

I'm not sure, as he moves south, that there wasn't a real barb in that last word. But I play along, angling my bottom for him, amazed that it just sits there, intact, when my old arse always seemed to ooze, and splay, and melt over the side of the bed, runny ganache down the side of a cake. Embarrassed, shy, feeling as though I'm on trial and am in danger of being returned, I do a bad impression of Dad's Army's Warden Hodges. 'Oi! Put that light out!'

Somehow, though, the joke falls as flat as my tummy. Somehow, being a funny woman when you're not fat or boss-eyed doesn't quite work. It is as if Keira Knightley just cracked a pun, then swore, when all she has to do is stand there, oozing icy beauty from every small pore.

He sits up. Takes another swig from his glass. His mouth is open. I can see his tonsils. A couple of dark fillings. He plants a dry kiss on the top of my head, as though he were a politician and I a child being proffered in a crowd. I try to fold my limbs alluringly, as though I am Robert Harbin, magicking origami shapes out of pieces of coloured card.

'What's wrong?' I ask him. Why am I always destined to play the diplomat? Someone should give me an embassy.

'Weeeell. It didn't help when we stopped at the petrol station you yelled at the woman, "Where's the baby? Where is it?"'

He has put on a stupid voice, mocking me. Bastard. I realise with a start he has put the old woman in a car with a faded pink sign in the back before me. Just as Neps put the taxi driver before me. Why does everyone come before me! Why am I always last? In the egg and spoon. In life.

I remember, now, she had taken ages to move from her spot. I was anxious and excited to get here and as her car was blocking our way, I noticed the faded pink sign in the back window: Baby on Board. So I'd muttered, 'That woman hasn't had a baby on board since 1982', and unfortunately, she'd heard. Any other couple would have laughed about this. But he had huffed and puffed and pulled away from the service station just on the wrong side of safely.

I say now, 'You weren't joking then, just now, were you, when you called me a bitch?'

'No,' he says sadly. 'I'm afraid I wasn't.'

. . .

199

We dress and go down to dinner. He tells me I look lovely; the dress is great and that I 'have the body for it'. Wow. I have the right body. Not the wrong body. Not someone else's body by mistake. It feels wonderful, after all the misery, the disappointment, the pain, the heartache, to be walking into a lovely restaurant on the arm of a handsome man. I have arrived. The eagle has landed. This is what I always wanted. I am normal.

We are a bit early, so we sit at the curved bar.

'What would you like?' the barman asks him.

'A Pernod, please.'

'And for you, Madame?'

I almost hiss 'Miss!' Patsy Stone fashion, but I just say, 'A glass of champagne, please.'

I wonder whether Jeremy shouldn't have ordered my drink first, but perhaps I am being old-fashioned. The drinks are brought and water added to the Pernod so it clouds. A bit like his mood.

'What's that French drink that is now banned?' I ask him. I notice his pupils are tiny black pinpricks. I must Google, later, what this means. Is he about to have a heart attack? Or is he simply on heroin? I read somewhere that if a man fancies you his pupils dilate, so why are his doing the opposite? Am I still that hideous?

'That's absinthe,' he says, ever the man of the world, and he clicks his fingers for the bartender, who comes over. 'Do you have absinthe, by any remote chance?'

A bottle is duly brought – of course they have it, this is Lime Wood – and a large schooner filled. It is viscous, bright green. Jeremy downs it in one. His face turns bright red. I often can't help but wonder how even when men are trying to impress they have little care or even awareness about how they look. It's as though they are above such trifles (mmm, I wonder if this place does trifle).

A few seconds later, we are summoned to our table. There are lots of couples, shiny and pink from a day by the pool. We sit down and I notice he wobbles slightly. Menus are brought. Now, Jeremy is coeliac, and because of this I have already warned the hotel, in a series of emails. I get a gorgeous basket of French sticks, while Jeremy is brought two slices of brown bread that looks worryingly like Warburtons.

'What's this?' he says, picking both slices up, sniffing them, almost using them as a flannel on his face.

'Don't do that,' I say. 'It's an Angela Hartnett restaurant. I chose it specially.' I wonder why all my special occasions are ruined. In a sandwich bar with a Skyr yogurt. In a five-star hotel, offered vintage beets harvested less than ten minutes ago in the walled kitchen garden. The only common denominator is me. Maybe it's me.

'Do what?' he says, slapping them down, scattering

cutlery. 'It's not white bread, is it? Why is your bread better than mine! And don't do that with your head.'

'What?'

'Look down. It gives you a double chin.'

He orders wine, and food. He wants the salmon and the John Dory but 'I'm not sure I can eat three courses. I'm not really that hungry'.

Important note to all mankind: if you are lucky enough to be taken to a Michelin-starred restaurant in a forest hotel by a woman for your Special Day, at least pretend to have an appetite. DO NOT turn your nose up. At least try to look grateful.

Our first courses arrive. He slings his crisp napkin onto the table.

'You think you're really special, don't you?' he says.

Where has this come from? 'Um. Yes, I do, actually,' I say. I don't, not really.

'You are a stuck-up – what's that rag you work for? Oh yes, Marie Claire – a stuck-up bitch with a real bloody attitude.'

I have no idea where this is coming from. Is he having a fit?

'You are an arsehole,' he continues. 'A dickhead. I don't trust you,' he says, shoving his plate away, pushing his chair back. 'You just want another sap to shell out for your children. Free childcare. Just like every other woman in the universe!'

The couple at the next table are starting to shift in their chairs. They probably saved for a year to be able to come here. How dare he ruin it for them.

It is as though nice Jeremy, kind Jeremy, has been replaced by a monster. A drooling throwback, like Sir Les Patterson. I suddenly realise Jeremy has had two mojitos by the pool, the large gin in the room, Pernod, the green whatever it was. A vat of wine. I try to calm him down. 'What do you want to do?' I ask him. I try to place a hand on his, but he bats it away. 'Go up to the room and lie down for a bit?'

He stands. He sways. He pushes his chair back and it falls with a clatter. 'Yes. I know exactly what I want to do. Let's go up to the room and FUCK!'

He says this to the Whole Room.

He disappears. Our untouched starters are taken away. I sip my champagne: try to stay cool. Try to stay cool. Our main courses arrive. The waitress, having witnessed the outburst, is as white as a sheet. His dead fish sits there, on its plate. Its eyes stare up at me. 'Please don't let me have died in vain,' it says. 'I used to have a family.'

Oh dear God. He's coming back. He slides into the banquette beside me. He misjudges his landing. Boof. Ow.

'You are a cunt, you know that? No wonder your gay husband couldn't stand you.'

How does he know that? How does he know he's

gay? They met, once, when Neps dropped the babies off, but that was barely two seconds. They barely spoke. Do men have a sixth sense? Was there a secret handshake?

'Fucking plastic surgery to make yourself perfect. Who could love that?'

'I think you should leave,' I say, gathering my napkin and my courage. I will myself not to cry. I keep my head down; ooh, no, head up. Don't want a double chin. I was normal when I came in, what, 20 minutes ago, and now I am part of some sordid Jeremy Kyle disaster. I didn't know scenes like this could happen to women who are a size 12, especially size 12 in a Victoria Beckham, which as all know comes up really gall bladder constricting fucking small.

And so, he does. He leaves. I toy with my pasta for a bit, but I can't stomach it. This, from someone who'd been known to lick the tablecloth. After what I think is a decent enough interval, I leave the table with as much dignity as I can muster and I creep up to the room. I open the door and to my relief all his stuff has gone: his holdall, his keys, his receipts and coins on the side, his washbag. My God, rooms are so much tidier without any male influence! I hang my little Do Not Disturb flag, then double-lock the door. Isn't it strange, that thing about men and relationships? One moment their penis is in your mouth. The next you are calling the cops.

I undo the dress, step out of it, hang it up carefully. I take off the stupid black bra, the thong, and change into my grey sweats. That's the best thing about getting dressed up to go on a date: taking it all off when you are back home. Even thin(ner), it feels good to peel off the artifice as well as the Laura Mercier corner lashes. To relax. Which I can never seem to do when there is a man in the room. I go into the bathroom to go to the loo. Eurgh. My feet are wet. I see little yellow droplets by the bowl. At the sink, tiny black specks of hair from when he shaved. God, men are disgusting. Even the handsome ones. It's as though we are expected to live with an alien. What was that song? I hate you so much right now.

I stare at my phone. A text from Neps, saying he hopes the mini-break is going well, and that the twins are tired and fast asleep. 'Oh, and I took the cat to the vet and he has cystitis! How is that possible? Is he a trans-cat?' I suddenly miss him. I wish he had been sweet, and funny, earlier. Or maybe he was and I was too busy and self-absorbed and chewing to notice.

And then a text from Jeremy. 'I can't abandon you here, so I will sleep in the car and drive you back in the morning.'

I reply: 'Don't bother. I will get the train.' Then I remember. It's my fucking car!

I was just settling down to self-medicate by watching

TV on my iPad when 'Bang! Bang! Bang! Bang!'

'Who is it?' I squeak improbably through the door. A really angry maid?

'It's me. I need my charger.'

I hunt around, find it plus his sunglasses, pants, toothbrush (why do all men need mothers? Why?), open the door a crack and hand them to him. 'You know I love you,' he says. He is actually swaying. 'I don't know what happened. I remember calling you a dickhead. When it is clear that I am the dickhead.'

'You're not driving while drunk,' I tell him.

'No. I will sleep in the car. Unless …'

I slam the door. Double-lock it. I stand there for a little bit, listening, but he has gone.

I manage to sleep. Next morning, I get up, shower, put on make-up in case he's lurking downstairs. I can't face breakfast, or the lunch I'd booked, so I check out, now nearly a grand worse off, and order a cab. The blonde receptionist, the same young woman who had checked us in only hours earlier, has the grace not to smirk, or say, 'Are you okay?' Or 'Jesus Christ, what on earth happened?'

I wait in the sun for the cab. Tall in my heels, skinny in my skinny jeans. People arrive and walk past me. Older men, greying (always), with slightly younger women (always), here for a romantic weekend. I see the men checking in checking me out. The women take me in

– the Paige jeans, the sheer Valentino, the heels, the Vuitton at my Essie Ballet Slippered toes – and I can swear they are jealous. They are painting onto me an imaginary life because of the way I look: how happy I must be. How loved. How free from worry and pain. The man in my life must be fetching the car, because someone this gorgeous is always cherished, looked after. Safe. I know they are doing this because I always did this.

I ask the driver whether we're headed to the right station to get me to London. He is eastern European, has an accent. 'Oh yes, platform 2. The ticket office is right there. You make sure you have a nice day.'

Isn't it telling how even a taxi driver is nicer to me than the man with whom I'm currently sharing a vagina.

As the train approaches Waterloo, I start to panic. Where should I go? Why is my life such a disaster, when I try so hard? Why are all those flabby women by the pool so happy and content, and I'm not? Why am I mired by conflict? Is it my fault? Am I really a horrible person?

And then a text from Jeremy. 'I am so sorry. I feel so ashamed. I now realise I have a drink problem. I really hope you can forgive me. Please come home.'

A few minutes later: 'Thinking further. You should not have to pay for the hotel when I ruined your stay. Can you send me the receipts and I will transfer you the money at the end of next week?'

He wants the receipts? He wants evidence? The man might come from a family who watch cricket and go wild swimming in rivers, but he clearly has no class.

Arriving at Waterloo, I join the queue for cabs. There are lots of couples, arriving in London for the weekend. I bet not one of them gets called a dickhead. After a few moments of indecision, I give the driver, already rolling his eyes at the stupid woman who can't remember where she lives, an address.

. . .

Fifteen minutes later, I am leaning on a buzzer outside Izzy's flat. A raven head leans out an upper window. 'Coo-ee!' she goes, waving her fag at me. 'Come on up! I've got drinkies!'

You see, this is why I love women. No miserable face. No arguments. No accusations. No silences. If I'd gone on a girly weekend with her, we'd have got drunk in the hot tub, weeing in the water, cackling loudly, not a care in the world. We'd have staggered down to dinner, still damp round the edges, linking arms, not caring who sees us. We'd have shared a delicious dessert with two spoons. She would never have flounced off before even the first course had had a chance to go cold. She would never have called me a dickhead.

'So, what's he done this time?'

I tell her. Every detail. I think at one point I make

little drawings. There is a graph, too. And a pie chart.

'I am shocked,' she says. 'God, when you said he started slurring his words, I thought you were about to say he had had a heart attack! What got into him? Is he jealous of you, being able to afford that stuff when he only ever went there on a freebie?'

I hadn't thought of that.

'No. I don't think so. But he has always drunk a bit too much, hasn't he? It's his culture. His parents always have gin in huge great bowls with peppercorns. He's never had to deny himself. Worry. Ooh … Maybe he was nervous?'

At this, she scoffs and her vodka spurts over me. 'Oooh, ow. That hurt coming out my nostrils. A waste, too. What are you going to do now?'

I tell her it's Friday afternoon and the twins are due at his flat after school. I can't confuse them, so I have to go back there. Face him. Act normal. 'He's probably got a hangover,' she says reasonably. 'He won't be up to going three rounds with you.'

And so I set off, again. Holding in not just my tummy but my emotions. But something is broken. There is a scar on our relationship. It is smarting. It's infected. It's oozing. It is about to come apart.

(A small note here, before we proceed. He never did transfer the cost of the ruined mini-break. He never mentioned it again.)

CHAPTER 13
Spoiled little rich-parented, public-school-educated, bicycling, yoga practising twat

Three months later

I'm in a cab, exhausted. I dropped my assistant Karis off first, because I'm not a complete and utter bitch, and anyway she is on the way from St Pancras International. I went to wave as she was unlocking her front door, but she was already talking into her phone, grinning broadly. All the lights in her house suddenly illuminated, just like that moment in The Towering Inferno when William Holden gives the order to 'turn on the lights on every floor!' Or Christmas on Oxford Street. How lovely, to be so festive just because your wife has returned from a two-day trip. The fact he is even awake is a good sign. She's a funny one, though. Loyal. Hard-working. But strangely ungrateful. Last Christmas, I gave her a Louis Vuitton traveller I'd been sent as a freebie. It must be worth £1,700, at least; they'd even monogrammed it in gold leaf with my initials. She'd accepted it and had taken it carefully out of its white cashmere bag, and looked pleased, and then she spied the initials. 'Oh dear,' she said. 'I will have to get that removed, or people will think I'm you.' There is no pleasing some people.

God, Paris is a shithole. Everyone is so rude! I must remember to ask the managing editor to book a different hotel next time: the Costes is so dark, I have to feel my way down to the lobby as though I'm Stevie Wonder. I do love, though, the fact that in the courtyard restaurant everyone still smokes, despite the ban. But now that Colette, where you could browse not just Chloé and Valentino but 100 different brands of water, has closed, there doesn't seem much point to being there; the Plaza Athénée opposite the Dior flagship would save so much time. The whole place, even the air, smells of Diptyque Ambre. Plus, it has a fantastic view of the Eiffel tower and a Dior spa where I can be renovated, like a dilapidated brownstone.

In the end, the cover shoot was a nightmare: I knew she would be a cow, just from the list of her required foodstuffs, faxed to me by her PR the night before, which stated she must be offered only 1% almond milk, wholegrain rice and kale, along with organic flat rainwater. When she arrived, three hours late, a mobile phone clamped to each tiny ear, and stripped down to her pants for our first fitting, she revealed the body of a six-year-old child. Nothing on the rails fit, as she has obviously shrunk since we shot her last: perhaps her record label put her in a hot wash by mistake. It will be the first time in history the magazine will be forced to airbrush on some extra flesh – smooth out that collarbone, those jutting ribs you could play like a xylophone – instead of excising spare tyres along with wrinkles, which is what we normally do. She refused to smile, too; I think the fact Patrick the photographer didn't know her name and asked for her new album – 'Ze racket!' – to be turned off didn't help. 'Ooo eez she? Ooo?'

I open the huge, heavy front door of the loft, manoeuvring my case, which is suddenly as heavy as a corpse. All the lights are off, of course they are. It would be far too much to ask him to leave a hall light on for once even if, like a toddler, he can't stay upright past 10 p.m. He is obsessed with getting enough sleep; thank the Lord the twins, the adults in this scenario, are with Neps. He didn't even call me once he knew I'd arrived at King's Cross, though I always track his plane in real time, so he has someone to talk to while he waits at the baggage carousel or queues for a cab.

I will unpack tomorrow; I can't possibly do it in the dark. Plus, I will wake him up. I peek into the bedroom. He is ostentatiously wearing a huge black eye mask. The blackout blinds are down. Whale song is playing. He really is a total dick sometimes.

I get undressed, pull on a T-shirt and shorts and brush my teeth. I fetch a bottle of water from the fridge and in the light I notice the laptop on his desk. It's open and on, and as I can't be bothered to unsheathe my MacBook, and knowing that anyway it will make a huge big 'bong!' when I turn it on, I sit in his chair and summon his from its slumbers, just in case anyone has emailed me about an early meeting tomorrow, or a cancelled cover shoot, a knee waxing emergency, that sort of thing.

The screen comes to life, and there is his email queue, lit up in front of me, for all the world as though it is Christmas morning. Blimey, that's unusual. He normally guards his emails with his life. He says it is the only 'space' in his highly monitored life; which is strange, given the flat is 2,850 square feet, excluding terrace, and I work all the hours God sends.

It is all pretty boring, just emails from travel PRs beginning, inevitably, 'Dear ____'. Except at the top, in bold type, lurks one he hasn't read due to his sudden onset narcolepsy. It's from someone called Deidre F—. There is a little gold star next to her name, which means she is a VIP.

Hmmm. I wonder whether to open it. I drum my fingers on the desk and crane my neck towards the bedroom. If I do open it, he will know. There are no earlier emails from her I can snoop on, as they've all been concertina'd into this one unexploded bomb. Of course, it might not be a bomb. It might be that the dry-cleaning woman is letting him know his shirts are ready. But no. She's Bangladeshi. This bird sounds German. And the subject header is worrying me: it says simply 'Plans.' What plans?

I sit in a little pool of blue light and I ponder. There shouldn't be any secrets between us. But, well, everyone deserves some respect and privacy. I'd hate it if he read my credit card bill or knew how much I spend in Space NK, or saw what my skin looks like in the magnifying mirror, or what my nether regions look like without a Hollywood (grey).

Oh, sod it. I'm going in.

'Hi, Jez! Are you still coming to NYC with the Wicked Witch of the West? Hope so! But how will you get away? I have so much planned, so much to tell you. Can't wait to see you. Auf Wiedersehen. Your D, always. With peace + love + gratitude. x'.

At first, I can't believe what I'm reading. I actually do a double take. It must be a joke. I read it again. Then, I try to see it in a good light. Perhaps she doesn't mean the pre-Christmas stay at the Mercer I have planned, along with a room with a view of the Empire State and business class seats on Virgin. Perhaps there is some other Wicked Witch in his life. But I know he isn't going to NYC any time soon, except with me. Jeremy is always quiet at Christmas – the busiest time in the hotel and hospitality world, so no space for freebies – and so I'd invited him to come along, told him I will only be shooting for two days, max, and the rest of the time we could just hang, chill, go shopping, ice skating in Central Park or just sit in the bar atop the Mandarin Oriental and drink in the view.

Now, normally, he eschews coming along on my work trips, feeling like a third wheel. When he got back from reviewing a hotel in Udaipur two weeks ago for Condé Nast Traveller, thin and nervy beneath the tan, he'd said, with a strange look on his face when I'd mentioned the Mercer, 'I'm not sure I can face another long-haul trip. Plus, I really have to get back to my novel.'

I only just had to time think, 'Well, that's charming,' when, a couple of days later, he made a complete volte-face. Saying he'd love to come, that it would 'make a change to stay in a hotel and not have to upend the mattress and count bugs and semen stains'. That he's always wanted to stay downtown, especially just before Christmas. 'We can get the twins' presents.'

Ah. So, this is why. This is why he changed his mind. I should have seen it. He is as transparent as a floor-to-ceiling window.

But do you know what? I'm suddenly strong and fierce. There is no time for tears. I have to find corroborating evidence. I have to know everything. I don't want to look and read, but I am compelled to scroll down, see the complete exchange. And oh dear God, it has gone on for two weeks; the first one is dated the night he landed. 'Just in cab on the way home. Wish me luck.' There are dozens and dozens of them. Words swim before my eyes … 'I miss you' … 'I keep thinking about our room overlooking the lake, and waking up and seeing your face' … 'The black lentils were out of this world! And all the lanterns reflected in the lake' … 'You didn't take a picture of that cat, did you, by the bonfire?' … 'No, I haven't heard from the rest of the gang, but what a lovely group, we really must all meet up' … 'Have you landed, how are you? I can't wait to see you again' … 'We have to do this carefully, I can't risk losing my chance to finish my novel. If she kicks off, she will put me off concentrating' … To that last one she has replied, probably typing while on her knees, 'Yes, of course, you are an artist, you need tranquillity.' His last couple of missives to his mistress read as follows: 'I miss you … NYC here I come!' … 'No, she hasn't any idea, but then she's always so busy and wrapped up in herself, the miserable, cadaverous cow.'

And finally, two emails back, just after the one from

her that rather illiterately confuses 'your' with 'you're', comes the David Cassidy line I had been dreading all along.

'I think I love you …'

I feel sick. As though I have just gorged on a six-pack of cream doughnuts from Greggs. How can this be happening? I am not Two Ton Tessie, so life is supposed to be perfect. I have a gap at the top of my thighs so wide you could drive a Winnebago through it. I can fit a size 10 on a good day, depending on designer, and on bad days I'm a size 12. I no longer need a bra. I'm beach body ready, even in winter. I'm quite a cheap date, really, as I never want a starter or a dessert. I only have one glass of wine, which I weigh first. Other men look at me when we walk into a room. Mums pushing writhing toddlers with backs arched in temper scowl as I walk past on his arm. I never refuse sex, ever. I look after myself. I am the best I can be.

Oh my God, it's exhausting when I think of everything I go through to look this way – the exercise regime, the lotions and potions (perhaps that's why they think I'm a witch?), the painful procedures (have you ever had collagen in your lips?), the nostril waxing, the spa treatments, the endless bloody clothes shopping and always, always having to deny myself just in case it makes me revert. I read somewhere that you need fat in your diet so the synapses in your brain can function, otherwise you become depressed. Perhaps that's what has happened, which meant I wasn't enough fun for him. (I can't remember when we ever sat together, laughing, on a balcony, just doing nothing other than basking in each other's company, as these two fuckers have obviously been doing. As well as bathed in each other's company. I was always anxious to go out, or see something, or stay in, or go for dinner, or get back and unload the dishwasher, or for him to just look at me.) Maybe I didn't pay him enough attention as, being me, being perfect on the outside is such a full-time, all-consuming job. I did buy him a car, which, given his addiction to cycling, he just left on the kerb. He still has no idea how to open the bonnet; he has no concept you have to occasionally put oil in. But still, still, I don't deserve this. He could have said something. I would have tried to change.

Exhausted from reading the emails over and over again, I slump in the chair. I am tempted to either go to bed and say nothing or to empty a bucket of iced water on his stupid head, but I bide my time. I slowly get up, straighten. I need alcohol. I head to the fridge, uncork a bottle, willing it not to make a noise, and just glug straight from the neck. This is no time for scales or a glass. The alcohol hits my bloodstream and then my brain almost instantaneously: that's the great thing about being thin, it takes just one sip to send you tiddly. And reckless.

Emboldened, I start to search the apartment, using the tiny light on my phone. Nothing in his desk drawers. His phone is by the bed where it always is, so I can't look at that, yet, but I go through the pockets of his pea coat: nothing. Not even a condom or a Nectar card.

I creep into the bedroom and slowly slide open the Italian wardrobe. Bugger, I'd forgotten it lights up, but we're okay, he's wearing an eye mask, remember. I go to his side of the wardrobe: all pressed Smedley sweaters in rainbow colours, dozens of pairs of carefully folded vintage Levi's, row upon row of classic trainers (dear Lord, and he had the cheek to complain about my spending habits!). A drawer of Calvin Klein pants and neatly folded socks which, for some reason, make me feel a twinge of regret and sorrow. I feel sorry for him. If he has been doing all this, cheating on me, texting, plotting, it means he hasn't been happy.

I am about to slide everything shut when I think to rummage around at the bottom, at the back. And there, in the furthest corner of the wardrobe, is his Leica, the one I bought him the very first time he went to India. I remember now, too, in a flash of memory as vivid as a film trailer, that he'd made his full-nappy face when he unwrapped it. 'What's up?' I'd said, barely able to believe, after all my online research, that I'd bought the wrong model after all. That I'd made a mistake.

'It's just that it's really heavy. Remember, it will be 40 degrees out there and I will have this, round my neck. The strap's really wide, too. It will make me sweat. I really don't think I'm going to take it with me. Sorry.'

That was a warning siren, wasn't it? WEE! WEE! WEE! Ungrateful, spoiled little rich-parented, public-school-educated, yoga practising bicycling twat! That's where his confidence, his carelessness originated. Public school. Parents with money and a nice house. A circular drive. How lovely to have a safety net. Mum and I had grown up so close to falling and crashing onto concrete: no net, no bungee tape, no parachute. A single mum, on benefits, with a devastating illness. Dear God, how I'd been taken in by him. But then again, he'd been taken in my me. The Vuitton holdall that was a gift. The BMI that was achieved by knife. It's all surface but, like David Attenborough cooing over a pond skater, he couldn't help but be a little impressed.

Anyway, forget the past. That was then. This is now. Breathe. Calm. Despite his protests, he had taken this camera with him on his last trip to India, the one he is just back from. I make off with it, a lioness with a gazelle, back to the office and I turn it on. It makes a little murmur, some cogs turn, and I glance up again, afraid he might have heard. No, nothing. I enter its library and I scroll. I tear it limb from limb, rip off the fur and feast greedily on its warm insides.

View out of plane window of clouds. Queue at customs. Inside of taxi. Plants. Prow of boat. Plate of curry. Boring. Inside of auto rickshaw. Lake at night. Lake at day. Boring. Child. Hotel bed. Elephant.

And then. Here she is. Ta-dah! There is no shock, no surprise. All my life, I knew something awful was going to happen. Something bad. To prove to me how worthless I really am. I knew, right on time, that she was going to arrive.

She'd been waiting in the wings all this time, a prima ballerina, all creamy legs, leotard, long neck and neat bun, poised to teeter centre stage en pointe. All this time, while I felt I was safe, and happy, and settled, she was being conceived, born, learning to walk, going through puberty, passing whatever it is they pass in stupid American high schools, before finally arriving – what immaculate timing! – to pirouette onstage and steal my live-in boyfriend.

Isn't it incredible? Men are so lazy and stupid, so arrogant, so self-assured, they don't even bother to delete incriminating photographs they have taken while ostensibly working hard for our future, abroad. That's how little he thinks of me and the twins. He couldn't be arsed to use his thumb and press delete, delete, delete.

Here she is, on a balcony overlooking the shimmering lake at Udaipur. She has blonde hair, is wearing a bikini top and white shorts, her empty head thrown back. She is brown and confident looking, no make-up, the sort of posh girl who travels to India in Birkenstocks to tell indigenous people how to dig wells. There is no self-doubt on her face. None. Her parents probably told her over and over, 'You can be whatever you want to be!' While my mum's only wish for me was that I got to adulthood without being run over.

I remember, now, with a start, that I had called him while he was away. I usually don't bother him all the time, as I know if I'm needy it gets on his nerves, but I happened to be in LA at the Standard Hotel prior to a job styling Helen Mirren and suddenly there was a minor earthquake. I'd been typing on my laptop and my chair actually moved across the room. And so, terrified, and a bit excited I was somewhere dangerous for a change when he thinks my life is so cosseted and five star, I didn't text or email, I actually called him. Ring. Ring. Ring.

And he had picked up, and he had sounded … odd. Even when I said, 'I'm in an earthquake, I'm scared,' he had replied, disinterested, as though I were a PPI claim salesperson, 'I only have a minute.' At the time, I could have sworn he was with someone – there was just a thickening of the atmosphere around him, no actual voices – but of course I dismissed the self-doubt. He must love me, I'm perfect. He wants for nothing. But now of course I'm thinking, who says, 'I only have a minute' to the love of their life when they are thousands of miles away during a natural, life-threatening disaster? I realise now of course that he was with her. Oh God. And I put my head in my hands. It's like the moment I called Neps after surgery. The disinterest. The distraction. It's happening all over again. Except this time, it's not another man, it's another woman. Which right now I am thinking is even worse.

Because here she is, in all her creamy normalness, in bed. He has actually taken a close-up of her asleep in bed; I would stab him if he ever did that to me: I'd undoubtedly have my mouth open and be drooling. But her, oh dear me no, she looks perfect, posed. An athletic arm is slung on the white linen, the wrist covered with those leather bracelets and friendship beads. God, I hate this type of woman – horsey, and strapping, and red-faced, and beautiful in a Nordic, Kate Winslet sort of way; I bet she can sail yachts single-handed, and go rock climbing, and eat a three-course meal without blinking – even if they aren't sleeping with my cunting boyfriend.

And then, I am really sorry, but I can put it off no longer. I fetch a great big stainless-steel pan from the kitchen – Le Creuset, really cunting heavy – and fill it with water. Into this, I drop two large packets of ice.

I stagger with the pan into the bedroom. I am a little bit sad about the pillows, and the duvet, and the Conran pink bed linen, and I groan with the effort of lifting it above waist height, thanking the Lord for all those Pilates classes. But, oh God, the effort is worth it. The effect is better than I even imagined.

The black eye mask whooshes off – 'oof' – a rubber raft in a tsunami. The overlong hair is now upright and the mouth is open, taking in great big waves of cold water, as though he's being waterboarded. Which he should be.

'What the f …'

He sits, choking and spluttering, and fumbles for the bedside lamp and his phone.

The light goes on. The phone is lifted, an ineffectual tiny shield. And then he sees me. 'Oh,' he says, and arranges himself upright on the pillows, pushing the wet hair out of his eyes. And immediately I understand. He wanted me to find out. Saves him the bother of confessing. He is exhausted from all the lying, the Oscar-worthy lovemaking. He is tired. Of me.

I turn on my heel and leave him to grab a towel or a lawyer or whatever and I head back to stand next to his desk, on which I have placed the camera. Exhibit A.

He emerges in a baggy T-shirt and pyjamas, rubbing

at his head with a towel. I don't think he apologises or tries to explain himself, but I can't hear what he's saying as a great big express train is running through my ears. I tell him I am going to email her.

'No, no, you can't,' he says. 'Please don't. I won't see her again, I promise. She was just someone I met in India, nothing happened. We were going to compare photos in New York, nothing else. I will never email her again.'

'No, but I am going to email her. I saw her photos on your camera. Nothing happened? At least have the courtesy not to lie.'

I give him a hard shove out the way, so violent he actually stumbles and looks shocked. Good. I want him to feel shocked. I want him to know that I am tough, I am hard. Anyone who can have their insides sliced open and almost starve themselves to death could be in the SAS. Sod round-the-world sailing. I can walk on water. I could jog to the moon. And so, I start to type, elbowing him roughly out of the way every time he tries to get near and delete things.

Dear Deidre

What a stupid, stupid bloody name. I assume you are a German immigrant; did you arrive by boat? No wonder Jeremy was shouting at the ball the other day during an international, willing it to go your way. How deeply unpatriotic; he should be sent to an internment camp. Having Googled your company's website, I can see, too, below the photo of your stupid face, that you are a travel agent. I always thought he was intimidated by my high-flying, award-winning success, the chippy, low-earning bastard, and now I have proof! And telling him you are 'off to work out': has he not told you he finds my constant body maintenance boring? And you telling him that one day you 'want to work for a not-for-profit' is akin to admitting you have virulent herpes: how on earth would you pay for his extravagant, yoga-every-day, Smedley wearing, novel writing, loft living lifestyle?

What sort of woman are you anyway, that you can sleep with another woman's husband? Have you not heard of the MeToo movement or do the numerous studs in your ear make you deaf? Would you like it if a man cheated and lied to you, or your sister, or your mum, or your daughter, should you ever have one – but then again, perhaps you're already pregnant? Was that the plan all along, to ensnare him?

And why am I the Wicked Witch of the
West? I have been nothing but nice to
Jeremy. I have bent over backwards to make
him happy; literally, sometimes. What is so
wicked about buying him a car, or giving him
six months off his job so he could write his
'book', or letting him go off to Ibiza and India,
with pocket money supplied by yours truly
and a lift to the airport, to find himself? Bet
he never told you any of that, did he? No, no,
no. It would have been, 'Oh, poor me. I'm so
unsuccessful and put upon and bullied and
henpecked I need to spurt semen in another
woman's mouth just to make me feel good
about myself.'

You are the wicked one, surely. Why do you
think your 'plan' of having his cock in your
stupid baggy cunt having just vacated the
bed in the Mercer hotel room his girlfriend is
paying for is in any way a good idea? Or moral?
Who thinks that to do so could possibly be the
basis of a happy relationship? To have it formed
on lies, and subterfuge, and making someone
else unhappy? And, okay, I can understand if
he met someone else and fell head over Cuban
heels in love, but to lie about it? He's still lying,
right now, cowering next to me, when I have

the photos of you naked in bed in front of me, saying nothing happened!

Can you not get your own man, in the whole of New York City and the Baltic States? Or are you that unattractive and boring and unsuccessful and stupid you have to get someone second-hand? Someone who, let's face it, is having sex with you just to piss me off?

I press send. It makes a satisfying little sound: whoosh! Your email has been sent. I really want to kill someone right now. I could have typed worse. That was me being really nice. And I am going to not just press send, I am going to press charges. I am going to get her sacked. I am going to destroy her. I am going to post her fat face on Instagram with the caption: 'Don't let the friendship bracelets and the bare face and the not-for-profit ambitions fool you; this one's a freaking whore.' I'm going to post a photo of him on Instagram, too, with the caption: 'Missing. One boyfriend. Six foot two, wiry, posh, probably wearing a rugby shirt, has curly eyelashes. Last seen entering a German travel agent.'

There are an awkward few moments while we wait for a reply. I can tell, just by his posture, he is desperate to get back to bed in order to be up early for yoga. Even with our future on the line, all he can think about is his smelly blue rubber mat. An email returns, with the header: Read.

'Oh, she can read, can she?' I say, hands protecting the keyboard like a ninja warrior. 'Now there's a surprise.'

Another email appears. I open it slowly, as though it were a teeny tiny parcel left under the tree on Christmas Day.

'I assume this is Pamela,' she has typed. Wow, get you, Sherlock. I told you those American degrees aren't worth the paper they're written on.

'Jeremy told me when we first met in India that he was in an unhappy, unfulfilling relationship and that he wanted out. I have not "stolen" him from you. He is reaching out for a better life. But I can see you guys are having a complicated moment, so I would appreciate it if you could stop abusing and harassing me over email. Peace + love + gratitude. D.'

I'm abusing and harassing her! The low-foreheaded, caramel-highlighted, fucking illiterate bitch. I swivel, slowly, in the Eames chair, an insane, platinum-haired Bond villain, to face him. If only Neps hadn't kept the cat. He has the cheek to actually smirk. I am tempted to wipe it from his face but instead I am suddenly made of steel, a Jeff Koons rabbit. 'And you,' I say, unfurling myself to my full five foot eight. I poke him in his scrawny chest. 'I want you OUT. Out of this flat and out of my life.'

$8^1/_2$ STONE

CHAPTER 14
She's like the wind

So, today, just a few weeks to go before Christmas, I'm in the Mercer Hotel in Soho, downtown New York, opposite the Prada store (what is the point to Prada when you're single and cuckolded? You might as well shop in Next, or Bonmarché). On the work trip I'd manipulated into being the perfect mini-break for the two of us. Alone. Without you.

I didn't throw him out, that night I discovered he was cheating on me with Deidre. It was his flat, after all. But I don't know. It was like the mini-break at Lime Wood all over again. I was stranded with no way to get home. He had turned into a complete stranger. I started to wonder what it is about me that is so unlovable. Why am I not enough? I worried, too, that my life had become so chaotic. That can't be good for the twins. I have to make something work. I have to try. I have to find out what other women have that I don't. What am I doing wrong?

Am I missing a chromosome? A trick? While I was in a taxi to the plane this morning, Jeremy sent me a text. I will reproduce it here, though I'm sure he doesn't want me to. Tough.

'Pam. Chubs. I know you blame me. I fully accept that blame. I shouldn't have got close to someone while away trying to find myself in India. Worse, having got close to someone, I should have been straight with you and told you. As soon as I got back. If not before.

'But the thing is, I have felt smothered by your expectations. I am not ready to be a dad to someone else's children. I feel my space has been invaded by … stuff. I feel you put them first, which of course you should. Maybe I am not old enough to be with a divorcee who has children. It is all too messy, when you know I like order. You always seemed tired, when I needed your full attention. I needed you awake.

'But I am not totally to blame. You still carry around with you this belief that you are undesirable. There is the aura of a bigger woman around you. I know that is harsh, but it is true. It's as if I always have to appreciate you, marvel at how well you have done, when to be honest you having been overweight, then losing it all, has nothing to do with me. It is not my problem. I didn't force feed you chocolate bars. What do you want, now you are "normal"? A badge?'

'Fucking cunting arrogant arse.' Oh dear. I said this out loud. Ramanganathrata, my driver, looked worried. I carried on reading.

'I didn't intend to get on so well with Deidre, but she is just so uncomplicated. She didn't invade me. She is confident in her own skin, which I like. She was take it or leave it, so I decided to take it. This is probably the most you and I have spoken, on any deep sort of level, since we met. I know I have issues. I know I am lazy. I am probably untalented. But I do deserve to be loved. And so do you.'

When I got on the plane, I was crying so much they gave me an upgrade. 'Are you okay?' the air stewardess kept saying. 'Has someone died?'

'Yes. In a way.'

I sat in my (much bigger; really nice, actually) seat, unable to concentrate on a film. How can my life be such a mess when I have just always tried so hard? I am so nice to everyone. To my mum. To Neps. To Jeremy. To my children. Why is being nice no longer a passport to happiness? I don't get up every day and think, right, what's a really bad move? I have always tried to do the right thing. Why am I repeating what happened to my mum: I am now alone, bringing up children.

The air stewardess loitered near me, offering me an ice cream. I was tempted. Is this to be the next chapter, me getting fat again? I can't let that happen. I can't let food bring me down. I can't let a burger be my only friend, a crutch, an excuse. I have to summon the pain of surgery again in my mind in order to stop myself eating. No thanks, I told her. Can I just have some water? Oh God, am I going to be a bore for the rest of my life? Is that what turned Jeremy off? Another text from him. I had saved it at the airport, something to savour when I got on board:

'You know I want to be a dad one day. And you won't give me that.'

I almost laughed at this one. He is a joke, truly. One moment, he is too young to be a stepdad. The next, he wants children. Make your bleeding mind up. And he knows I can't do that, won't do that. What a cliché he is. Oh, how he is grasping at get-out-of-jail cards. I am well shot of him. Truly I am.

. . .

I will never get used to travelling alone. No one to heft your case onto the weighing thing at check-in; the plastered-with-make-up woman from Virgin will never think to do it, so busy is she staring at her screen and typing with her acrylic nails, completely uninterested in a female passenger. No one to go and peer at the board for the gate announcement while you finish your coffee. No one to help find your seat and give you theirs, next to the window. No one to stick their hand up for your special meal. No one to lift your bag into the locker. No one to chat to. No one with a shoulder to lean on. No one to help find the right luggage carousel or a cab. And now here I am at the reception desk of the Mercer Hotel: it is all white and floaty, as though I'm in heaven. Here I am, in this lovely place; I am thin, sort of, but still I am not happy. Turns out I should have not just sworn off Walnut Whips. I should have sworn of men.

'Hey, Mrs —. Welcome back! We have a lovely deluxe room for two, and two room keys, and two terry dressing gowns. Will you be requiring a dinner reservation for two?'

Another fucking patronising low-earning bastard. Could he have said the word 'two' more often?

'Um, it's just me, I'm afraid. What can I say? I still have cellulite. So just one room key, thanks. And I will be having dinner in my room. Alone.'

Of course, these people don't give two hoots that I'm on my own. They wouldn't care if I arrived with a turkey as my emotional support animal or if I had no legs, let alone no husband. I am nothing to them. Just another vaguely warm body in a small, expensive postage stamp of New York space.

. . .

Having got my work done in record time – a shoot in Grand Central Station, another shoot below a Christmas tree in some other godawful place – I was now at a loose end before my flight home. No husband to pander to. No one to go out for dinner with. I mean, who wants to go skating in Central Park … on your own; I expect, as in all London parks these days, you'd get arrested unless you had a child or a boyfriend in tow. And so, with all this free time, I hatched a rather cunning plan.

I looked up the location of the whore's office – a lovely building, actually, not far from Barneys and the Apple store, so quite convenient – and I came up with a ruse. I would take along a package, ring the buzzer downstairs and pretend to deliver it, asking the probably moronic lump on reception for 'a photo ID and a signature'. And, of course, out she would emerge on her little trotters. And I would confront her face to smug, German, boyfriend stealing face. After that? Well, I'm not sure. I consider disfiguring her. Giving her a bill for moving out.

It all goes surprisingly well. I have a box – a dreadful Christmas gift that had been couriered to my hotel by Donna Karan: bed linen, awful stuff, something from her diffusion line – and so I've scratched off my name and written hers instead. I am looking, in my opinion, my absolute best. You know that moment when the mouse that is Anne Hathaway puts on some Chanel and gets a new haircut in The Devil Wears Prada? This is like that moment. I have been to the Bliss spa around the corner for an oxygen facial. I'm wearing a black Moncler jacket, pipe cleaner jeans and biker boots. Every tiny pore is exuding English class and the fact my grandfather fought the Nazis in the war; I am going to bring up this fact in conversation.

I'm slightly nervous, but I figure I have nothing to lose, bar my liberty if she gets me arrested; at this point, I figure prison is worth it. (I wonder if they allow waxing in prison, and tweezers.) I arrive at her building (I walked all the way from downtown, so have a glow). I crane my neck to take in the building's height and feel giddy. I spot the name of her company on the long list in the marble lobby. I press the buzzer. I get in the elevator and I glide, clutching my box and my dignity. I am disgorged into a white reception area, with plants and water and art on the walls and white designer chairs. I go up to the desk and I say her name, which makes it all rather thrillingly real. I tell the young woman, who is already looking wide-eyed and scared, that I have a package for her. She is dubious, as I don't remotely resemble a courier. I tell her I am from Donna Karan, so she bows her empty head and she presses the button: beeep!

After a few moments, there is a 'click, click, click,' and there she is. She looks different from the screen on the camera, from the hot innards of that deer: not post-coital, for one. Dressed, too. Now, there's a surprise. She actually owns clothes.

'Can I help you?'

I put down the package and extend a gloriously brown, skinny hand. I no longer wear my wedding and engagement rings. They became too big and currently reside in a box in my chest of drawers.

'Deidre?'

'Yes.'

'I believe you've been fucking my boyfriend.'

And oh dear God, all hell breaks loose. You'd think it was Watts, in the sixties. Or Compton, in the nineties. Great big uniformed men are suddenly surrounding me while Deidre, who is not as stunning in person – is quite ordinary, in fact, and well covered, and short, and stupid looking – looks on, alarmed.

'If anyone should be arrested, it's her!' I say, pointing at Deidre.

The big men stop, and Deidre, obviously not wanting to be sacked or tasered, pulls on a coat – caramel Max Mara; never accuse me of not knowing my labels. And how much do junior travel agents earn these days, anyway, if they can afford that? – and flicks her honeyed locks from under the collar, grabs her phone and what is left of her dignity and we are off. She pretty much bustles me into the lift. It is awkward, not just because I am still holding quite a big cardboard box – I am also being squished in a small space with a woman who barely three weeks ago was enjoying cunnilingus from my soulmate. I wonder if we should compare notes: 'Did he do that thing of getting you on your side, spooning behind you, then pushing you really hard in the back, so your body folds in half like a clam, and your head is as far away from him as possible, your arse exposed and at exactly the right angle?'

'Um, no, he never did that.'

We exit via the revolving door – I wait for my own little Chocolate Orange segment of space; I still have my pride if not my live-in partner – and she strides off down the avenue at top speed, scattering tourists who have dared to come to her city and get in her way. I scuttle along behind, clutching my thin coat around my thin body. What was that Dirty Dancing song? She's like the wind. I bet she goes up Everest at this speed, barking at Sherpas about the best route. She's so confident, such a know-all. Even when she realised it was me in reception she wasn't fazed. She didn't try to hide. She just brazened it out. She disappears inside a vegan cafe and I follow. Everyone waves at her, smiles or nods. My God, she's popular. When I enter a cafe, people hide and throw tea towels over things.

'What do you want?' she asks me, unravelling a scarf from around her neck like a magician.

'Um, for you to die and for my boyfriend to come back to me?'

I don't really say this. I um and ah and squint at the blackboard. 'A double espresso, please.'

I sit down, hanging my coat ostentatiously on the back of the chair. I want her to see my arms. She returns. Her cheeks are as ruddy as Tess of the fucking D'Urbervilles'.

'That was quite a shock, that you would actually come to my office, my place of work,' she says, sipping something clear and cold: water.

'Yeah, well, what did you expect? And not nearly as shocking as me having to find photos of you naked on his camera. And read your frankly shocking emails.'

'Yeah, he should have told you. He said he was going to, as soon as he got back to England, in person. And then he said he had told you, so that was why we planned to meet up in New York.'

'Bit odd, bringing me along, like a beard or his social worker. Where did you imagine he'd be sleeping?'

'Oh, well, he said he already had a flight booked with you, so it was a shame to waste it. Of course, he wasn't going to be with you, in your hotel.'

This doesn't add up. She had written, 'How will you get away …'

An image of Mrs Richards flies unbidden into my brain: 'You lying hound.' But I let this slide.

'So, how did you meet?'

She has the gall to start smiling at the memory. 'We were just at a sacred site, both climbing up these hundreds of steps, most of which had worn away. I lost my footing, then I was surrounded by all these children begging for money. So, he rescued me, sort of.'

And then? 'We decided to travel together for a bit, pool resources and knowledge [bodily fluids, more like]. There were places and things he wanted to show me. The lake, for one. The palaces. Oh, and the Golden Temple.'

Oh, and his golden penis.

'So, you started sleeping together.'

For the first time, she actually has the decency to look uncomfortable. 'He told me he was living with someone, a mum.' She almost spits that last word. I wonder she can even say it. 'It was obvious, anyway, as you kept phoning and texting. [What? That's a lie, for a start.] But by the second week, he said he realised he wanted to be with me. That your relationship had long been over. That he'd made a mistake, felt sorry for you. He's done it before, you know.'

'What?' I can feel my heart, beating in my chest. The train is back, in my ears. What has he done before? Macramé? Scuba diving?

'Had an affair. Someone called Jess? There was a yoga teacher, too, at some point, he thought he was in love with. And an older woman, a famous journalist, coke addict: his supplier, I think.'

Oh, great. This all just gets better and better. Carry on, why don't you? He never loved me. He's a sex addict. He's a junkie. I don't want to hear any more, but I can't help it. Now I'm the addict, wanting one more fix, even though I know it might kill me. I'm my old self, my big self, thinking, well, there is one last Malteser rolling around in the box, so I might as well chomp on it. How much worse can it really get? I realise I am grasping on to her, a Max Mara-clad raft in the wreckage of my love life, trying to find the little black box that will tell me why it all went so horribly wrong.

'So why did he ask me to move in if he was already sleeping with other women?'

'Like any man, I suppose: he wanted security, a nice, easy life. He settled.'

Yeah, my contacts in the media world. My discount cards. My beauty: an ornament or a pot to plant his ambition in.

'So, he never loved me. Never fancied me.'

'I'm not your therapist,' she says, somewhat nastily.

I wonder how she can possibly know he will not do the same thing to her, and then the thought occurs to me. It arrives, an inflatable raft after that plane crash, all brightly lit and bobbing, that they might not even be together anymore. I hold the thought in my head, clinging to it like one of those white polystyrene floats, just for a few seconds: she must realise he is a serial cheater, he can never commit, he is weak, he can never be trusted, that he lies all the time, and so I ask her:

'Are you still seeing each other? Are you still, you know, together?'

I can see her thinking, hmm, should I lie? Does she have a gun? And then she decides, nah, and drops another bomb. The shock is so great droplets of espresso land on the table, and on my face and hands.

'Well. After you found the emails and the photos, I ignored him for a few days. I didn't want to get in the middle of you guys and your pain. And then he called me. Told me he hadn't had the heart to say he was in love with someone else because when he'd got home from Heathrow you'd seemed so frail; he told me a little bit about your psychiatric problems. The surgery. The dramatic weight loss. He was worried what you might do. But when you found out. Well. We actually met up in London.'

Oh. My. God.

. . .

I remember after Emailgate, a few days later, I was woken, at the crack of dawn, by the sight of him pulling on his best cardigan, the Burberry one I gave him, and hopping around, pulling on shoes. I could have left, I suppose, but that would have been defeatist: a break-up so soon after the last one. I still loved him. Wanted him. Most of all, I didn't want the surgery and the weight loss to have been in vain.

'I didn't want to wake you or the babies,' he said.

'Where on earth are you going?' It was too early for yoga and he wasn't in stretchy Lycra and a John Travolta sweatband.

'Oh, a mate I met in Kerala is on a stopover, on the way back to Canada. I said we'd have a few beers.'

'But it's six in the morning.'

'I know, not now. I will call you later. I do love you, Chubby.'

Chubby is his non-ironic name for me. He had come along to one of my psychotherapy sessions, when the not eating had taken over after me and Neps broke up and the sorrow of my broken marriage had broken me, and he and the therapist had got along like a house on fire. I might as well have not even been in the room; I should have just gone shopping in South Molton Street. Jeremy was praised when he said he just ignored my whining, cooked whatever he fancied, went off and did his own thing with yoga and work and meeting his friends, as most important of all he was not being 'an enabler'. So, being kind and thoughtful and caring and looking after a woman is somehow 'enabling' our craziness. Hence: Chubby.

But that early December morning? I should have known. I should have listened to my instincts. I should have listened to my gut: it might be small, but it is still quite vocal. He was going to meet her.

. . .

Back to the dreaded Deidre. I ask her what day it was: her layover (leg-over), when exactly had they met up? She has a think. I'm tempted to shine the light from my phone in her eyes. She says she can't remember. I tell her to look at her calendar and at last she looks at her phone and tells me, and it all suddenly makes complete sense. Of course, he was meeting her. In the cashmere cardigan I bought him.

'So, is he here, in New York?' I'm suddenly worried he is going to appear, that he took the flight after all, wearing a baseball cap, and that I am going to see him. I so want to see him. I straighten in my chair at the prospect. There are butterflies in my empty stomach.

'Oh no, he's not moving here. I am going there to be with him. I'm moving into his flat!'

Ah. Now I understand the phone call. I'd been coming out of the Royal Opera House, two days before this trip, and he had called me. 'I need to talk to you about the apartment,' he'd said.

'Can we not speak when I get back home?'

'I don't want conflict, I just don't need it. [God, now he sounds like a woman. Maybe I'm a lesbian after all.] I need to ask you now.'

Fearing the worst, a battle, a sleeping bag on Piccadilly Circus (I've spent so long worrying about whether my upper arms waggle, I haven't even thought about securing my own financial future or real estate. Ah. So maybe that is why men want us to worry about our bodies. They know we will be less on the ball when it comes to divvying up our assets), I simply replied: 'Jeremy. Just do what you think is morally right.'

'Okay. Thing is, I really need you to move out. You can go back to the house in Brixton. Throw whatshisname out. I'm afraid it's really not my problem.'

I turn my attention back to her. I can see by the way she is shifting in her seat she wants to leave and is also desperate to look at her text messages. She is resisting, as she can probably tell I am poised to wrestle it from her cheating hands to read his missives.

. . .

When I got back from New York, I told the taxi driver to take me to the flat. As I placed the key in the door, I half expected him to have changed the locks. Or moved. But no, it was fine. I could still get in. He's not quite that churlish.

He was in the kitchen, leaning on the island. He had

a glass of something clear next to him. Vodka, probably. Well, everyone needs a prop. Food was mine. Booze is his. We all have our drug of choice. The difference is we overeaters don't have the side effect that means children are trafficked in South America. We don't start beating people up in the street after one too many Mr Whippys. Well, I might, I suppose. If they got on my nerves and threatened to nick my cornet.

'I hear you turned up at Deidre's workplace,' he said. His voice as well as his glass was full of ice. 'Was that really necessary? She has nothing to do with this. She is very upset.'

'She's upset? Oh dear. Poor put-upon Deidre. Tell her to go meditate. You told me you loved me. You asked me to move in with you. You knew I had been hurt, betrayed. You promised never to do that to me. What was it you wrote in that card? "Let's have a lovely evening, and an even lovelier life together." Why would you write that if you didn't mean it? Do you know what it is like to have your husband leave you for another man?'

'No. Obviously I don't. But I am sure you are going to tell me.'

I am, actually. At length. 'I felt worthless. Hideous. To blame. You put me back together again. You got me. Not just my jokes, but my fragility. I helped you, too.'

'When?' He took another huge swig.

The cunting fucking bicycling bastard.

249

'Okay. Here's just one example. Remember when you had to write that column for The Sunday Times, and they'd returned it, saying it needed a, and I quote, "lightness of touch". I added a few jokes.'

He just looked down. I was on a roll now.

'I paid for stuff, so you could write your book. When have you supported my work? When I told you the Mail wanted a piece after the shows at London Fashion Week on skinny models, and I was excited to be asked but scared as I had only 20 minutes before filing, you know what you replied?'

'I have no idea. I am sure you are going to enlighten me given you have the memory, if not the girth anymore, of an elephant.'

'You said, "Fuck 'em." How is that helpful? How is that supportive? Because you were so spoiled, you have no work ethic. Well, do you know what, I hope old Droopy Drawers does come here, to live.'

He looked shocked that I knew this. She obviously didn't fill him in that she had let that slip. I could see his brain going, 'Why did Deidre tell her that? Is there no solidarity these days among couples who love each other?'

I carried on. 'Because she won't be easy. She's from New York. She is entitled. She says things like peace + love + gratitude. She will soon get pregnant, give up work, stay in bed all day, and then where will you be?'

'I will take my chances.'

And those are the last words I ever hear him speak.

. . .

One year later

I am still a little bit fat. What with all the hoo-ha of moving back to Brixton, I started to eat again, just a little, just to keep my energy levels and my spirits up. Nothing extreme, not like before. But I no longer eat just half a banana, placing the bottom in a cup for later. I chomp on the whole thing. Because what is the point? Being hungry didn't make a man love me. I was supposed to ask Neps to leave. He did offer, after all, that first morning I arrived with all my bags in the hallway, in a New York state of mind: i.e. insanely angry.

'I can go and stay at my parents',' he said.

'Do they still blame me?' I asked him.

'For what?'

'For the divorce. The marriage breaking up. Me moving in with the alcoholic drug addict.'

He looks surprised, goes to say something, then just decides to carry on. 'Oh, no. I told them. I told them we broke up because I'm gay, that none of it was your fault. That I had made you live a lie. That I put your health at risk.'

Blimey. This is all news to me. Why on earth didn't he tell me they were okay with it all? It turns out his parents were surprisingly supportive and understanding. When his sister came round later that day to take the twins out, give us a break while I sorted myself out, so we could talk, I took great pleasure when she grilled me in the kitchen about her brother's new boyfriend, in telling her that the new man is 'like, white, white'.

We talked, and eventually we decided that, yes, it would be best if he went to his parents' for a bit. 'Are you not ready to move in with him, the Ginger Biscuit?'

He laughed. 'Not yet. We are taking things slowly. I don't want to get into another situation where I promise everything and then leave. He isn't a bad person, you know.'

'Really?'

'No. He was the one always telling me I should tell you. That it wasn't fair on you. I was the one who was always too scared.'

CHAPTER 15

Why are women taught only to make cloth clothes peg holders, not how to build a life?

I was listening to Radio 4 the other day, as you do. It was a documentary about how humans first became monogamous. It turns out it doesn't come naturally to us, as I am in no doubt you are not surprised to hear. It was all to do with when people stopped being hunter-gatherers, always on the move, and started to become landowners. Men wanted to know they were handing their land and houses onto their own children, so they stuck around. That is all it is. That is what every Jane Eyre novel and Richard Curtis romcom movie is built upon: inheritance. Stamp duty. Walls. Circular drives. Not love, not really. Continuity. Ownership.

And then I read a piece somewhere – or was it a book? I can't remember – about how the sixties didn't really liberate women at all. That it was a lie. That decade, of the Beatles and the Mammas and the

Pappas and Twiggy and David Bailey, with its free love and not-so-free drugs, mainly, if not exclusively, benefitted men. Until that point, if a man wanted to have sex with a woman, he had to marry her. In return for all that sex, he looked after her. Went out to work, while she made a home and brought up the children. That was the deal. Come the summer of love, women just gave it up, willingly, and men took it, eagerly. They couldn't believe their luck. They no longer had to marry her and support her and her children and put up with her moods or dig in their pockets. They could move on. Women's lives became less stable, less predictable: precarious. There was no status quo. No deal. No pact.

In the fifties, women were constrained and judged by domesticity: how clean their house was, how ironed their children's clothes, how perfect their home-cooked meals, how snowy their front doorstep. It was a marketeer's dream. By peddling this dream, he could sell fridge-freezers, Hoovers, washing machines and laundry powder. Women escaped the marketeer's clutches for a bit, in the sixties. We made our own clothes. A sixties mini pinafore using a Butterick pattern was easy and cheap to run up. There was a pressure to be thin, and leggy, and flat-chested, but that look was only meant to last three or four years, before the maxi and adulthood set in. Women weren't meant to resemble children for very long. They were still meant to grow up, have children, wear decent skirts to the knee. Eat carbs.

But when I came of age in the nineties, everything had changed. We were no longer exclusively sold stuff to make our homes better. Instead, we were sold stuff to improve and renovate and polish ourselves. Not just eye gel, and night cream, and day cream, and pore strips, and décolletage cream, and corner lashes, and bath gel, and exfoliating scrubs, and so-called spa treatments, in a so-called spa that is really a bath tub in a corner of a room and underqualified, underpaid children as therapists, and gym membership, but Fendi baguettes, and logos, and shoes that were suddenly classified as 'art', although what these shoes were trying to say, other than 'I can't do steps. My feet hurt,' I have no idea. That skinny ideal, not meant to last very long, became entrenched. Suddenly, women were supposed to stay slim, and supple, and young, and raven-haired, and smooth-skinned, forever. That's the ultimate oppression, I think, the one that dictates we should stay girly forever. Expected to be beach body ready not just in snow, but well into our nineties. I sometimes wonder if, when I'm 70 years old without a pension or a home or a man, I will still be forming my limbs into a pretzel for my next extreme bikini wax.

And food. Oh, please, dear Lord. Don't get me started on food. The reason women stopped cooking was because we had bought all the appliances we could possibly need and we were having to work all the hours God sends in order to pay for all this stuff, not to mention because our husbands had left us, and so we started buying little rectangles of gloop we could put in the microwave because we were so exhausted and – did I mention this? – our husbands had left us. We ordered food online, just so we could spend more time with our 'families', whom we were slowly poisoning while they increasingly ignored us, glued as they are to screens. I don't blame anyone who says she doesn't have time to cook. My God, all those TV cooking shows, where a three-course meal takes 15 minutes, are all lies, smoke and mirrors: no one films the blasted celebrity chef doing the shopping, the queuing, the trying to work out how the self-checkout works ('Place the item in the bagging area'; 'Why don't you shut the fuck up!'), the lugging of carrier bags until our fingers turn red, the unpacking, the loading of the dishwasher, the unloading of the dishwasher! This is the modern woman's burden: making fantasy into reality while not complaining. No wonder we are either too fat or too thin. Too cramped by other people or too alone. Too angry. Too disappointed.

But when you have a problem with your size, everyone says, well, you should simply eat less: calories in, calories out. If you are anorexic, you are told to just put something in your mouth, chew and swallow. You do not have cancer. You can get better. How hard can it be?

But I know my relationship with food – such a simple thing, isn't it? Flour and broccoli florets. Little triangles of Happy Cow cheese. Penguins. Frozen peas. Not scary at all. Inert little objects that have no real power over us – led me down the path which has meant I have been abandoned, used and ultimately cast aside by two outwardly very different men. I was so apologetic about being fat, I married a gay man. I was so thrilled with the novelty of being able to fit inside a body-con dress without oozing out over the edges I didn't notice my new boyfriend didn't love me or even like me that much. And who turned out to be a self-obsessed, narcissistic, untalented drunk (bitter, moi?). He said he wanted a woman who loved herself. Who could 'live in the moment'? Not worry about tomorrow. Who was confident. What he meant was he needed a woman who was a bleeding, self-deluding idiot. Problem is, I was too needy, too nervous, too self-doubting for both of them. I can see that now. They were the problem. Not me at all.

I wonder there aren't classes in school that teach you all this stuff, to keep you sane and solvent and happy. Not just classes in how to choose the best mortgage and credit card, but classes in how to choose the best life. How not to be duped. The signs to look out for. Wouldn't a class entitled 'Signs your boyfriend is having sex with other women and taking coke' or 'Signs your husband is having sex both ways with a man with a ginger beard' be SO much more useful than a geography field trip to sketch truncated spurs in Norfolk or an outing to see Henry IV Part One at the Globe? Rather than a domestic science lesson in how to make cheesy potatoes and fashion a cloth peg holder for your washing line (I swear to you, I was taught both of those things, at extreme and tortuous length; I actually embroidered my cloth bag with little items of clothing), wouldn't a class in how to keep your home if your husband turns out to be banging another man be more apt? Or how to deal with an unfair boss who pays you less than a man doing your exact same job, but badly and with less imagination? Or how to deal with social services when your mum's care plan is rejected, the hours of her carers snipped in two? How to deal with officialdom, and HMRC, sexists and bullies at work, and bank managers, and builders, and EDF, and car mechanics, and sniffy little shop assistants, and all those people who only care about their own happiness, not yours.

The ultimate marketeer's wet dream of course is to sell women the idea – the fantasy – of romantic love. Our economy is built on this rubbish. Not just the film industry, magazines, fiction, Boots (dear God I hate Boots so much right now; 'Do you have a Boots loyalty card?' says the robot by the till, who peddles Kit Kats along with colostomy bags. 'No, I shop here as infrequently as I possibly can,' is my usual reply when I'm buying hair dye and collecting Mum's prescription), Topshop and wedding venues ('Still a private Georgian estate, this family home can be all yours for the day, as long as you stump up 20 grand and don't complain about the creaking floorboards and the crows pecking at flies at your window at 6 a.m., and you vacate the property by 10 a.m.'), but the property market as well; dear God, doesn't everyone bar you get a boost when you get divorced and it all goes tits up? Solicitors, when you hire them to divvy up the goods. Estate agents. Therapists. Removal men. Leg waxing beauticians. Spas, viz, 'A natural and holistic menu of treatments by …' Oh, shut the fuck up. He will cheat on me with a man I guarantee has pubic hair. He will cheat on me with a woman with no self-awareness at all.

My whole mission in life was to try to be perfect. To be the desired size as prescribed by the (mostly) men who decided, due to economics, profit, speed and lack of expertise, that the ideal shape was to be pretty much straight up and down, as of course such things as darts (the triangular things in dresses, not the speary things you throw in a pub), and structure, and good quality fabric cost money. That is why we hate ourselves. Profit. Greed. And certainly not our greed for tiramisu or sticky toffee pudding.

I wonder why we buy (literally) into all this stuff so readily. It can't just be because we want an orgasm. I climax far more quickly when a man is not in the room at all. It can't be for financial stability, as shown by the fact I married a teacher with a penchant for designer trainers. It can't be for map reading, not any longer: we have Google maps, or a nicely spoken Satnav Lady who calmly talks us down to our destination without flying into a temper. It can't be for mowing the lawn or putting up pictures, as men these days have lost these skills, as surely as I no longer know how to make my own bread. It can't be for making us laugh. I'm sorry, but I have yet to meet a man who makes me laugh out loud, bar Basil Fawlty. Real men aren't funny, are they? Or am I just moving in the wrong circles.

I don't want my son or my daughter to grow up as I have: apologetic. Worried. Always in a rush, and for what? What exactly do we think we are late for? I don't want either of them to get married, be lumbered with children who, let's face it, mean you are on red alert for the next 30 years, unless you die first. God, even Prince Harry is now saying the optimum number of children per couple if the planet is to survive is two. The only lesson I want my kids to learn is one of confidence. Self-acceptance. To have a passion outside of themselves, so their own well-being becomes secondary, almost: medicine (veterinary, preferably, given we have a now quite elderly cat), or painting, or poetry. Cycling to see the world, not burn off calories. Singing. Opera. That would be nice. So much more calming and uplifting than weighing coriander. How stupid and pointless is that.

. . .

Neps is right, in a way. Worrying about how much you weigh, how much space you take up on this planet, whether you are a size 38 or 40 in Italian designers, are merely a white woman's problems, when others in the world have so little. Counting calories is the modern-day equivalent of wearing the hobble skirt, or foot binding. We need to stop dreaming of goals. They swiftly become gaols.

8¹/₂ STONE

CHAPTER 16

*In the words of the great seventies prog
rock band Free: It's all right now. Sort of...*

One year later

Tonight is Christmas Eve. I did a Click and Collect
order from M&S back in October. I have bought the
twins presents: bicycles! I know, I really, really hate
bicycles when peddled by adult men, but they are my
subtle way of getting them up off the sofa and away
from their tablets and out in the fresh(ish) air. I am not
going to make them paranoid about food, because as
we all know, that pendulum can swing either way. I am
going to tell them, Christina Aguilera-fashion, that
they are beautiful, in every single way, every single day
of their lives. But I want them to be healthy.

And, of course, I have invited Mum. Not just for
Christmas, and I haven't told her this bit yet, but, like
a brand-new puppy, she is to move in with us for
life; I'm just hoping for a bit less wee and slightly less
chewing. I've ordered a sofa bed on the never-never

for the sitting room, plus I've looked into how much it would cost to add a walk-in shower to the downstairs loo, proper safety railings and a ramp to the back door.

I don't know if there was a moment when I knew I didn't need any of them: not the gay husband. Not the stupid, spoiled, miserable prick of a boyfriend whom I have no doubt will move from one woman to the next, grazing on them, sucking them dry, like a hummingbird flitting from flower to flower, only far less attractive and cheerful and busy. But now I know I can make a man desire me I seem no longer to want it. All that angst and longing, when the reality is it is too easy, really, to make a man want you. Just a bit of artifice. You don't even have to be interesting, or funny. Dear God. The dreaded Deidre proved that, the boring cunt.

I did have one revelatory moment, driving at last back to my little house when I left Jeremy for the last time, after Emailgate. Neps, when I had called and sobbed to him between great big gulps that hurt my throat down the phone about the dreaded Deidre, told me he was going out to be with Ginger Beard Man to give me some space; the twins were at school, and so I knew the place would be empty. I turned the radio up high, and Meghan Trainor was singing 'All About That Bass'. I started bopping along to it. I felt happy. Wow. That's new. I remember being happy, when I was a child. When all I had to worry about was whether or not I got home in time to watch Magpie.

In a queue on Vauxhall Bridge over the Thames, other drivers noticed me and they started to smile, too. Why was I never this happy as a teenager? Why did I waste all those years being miserable? Why did I think having a boyfriend is all there is to life? Then, when you've got him, you have to hang onto him! There is so much more. Telly. I love TV! Girlfriends: just going out and getting the giggles. Wetting yourself with laughter; I've never, ever done that with a man. I have always been en garde! Wary. Not laughing too much in case it made my face look hideous or gave me lines. Who exactly imprisoned us in this world where we are only judged by our BMI and the things we own? They don't make us happy. My God, in his bloody loft I was always carrying round a coaster, scared to leave a mark. Today, now, I'm happy. All that wellness rubbish is right about one thing: you have to learn to live in the moment. Stopping at the traffic lights, a young man on a bicycle peered into my car. Drawn by the music, like a moth to a flame. 'Really beautiful face,' he said.

'Yeah,' I told him, putting the car in first. 'The rest of me's not bad either.'

And so it was, two months before the office broke up for Christmas, I went into the brittle blonde's office with a mock-up of a new cover for our January issue. Of course, for the last million years, the cover line has always been, 'New Year, New You!' With that beach ready body on the cover. Airbrushed, elongated, hairless, impossible. Even the models don't look like that. Even Bella Hadid probably has thread veins and orange-peel skin. Even she will grow old. One day.

But not this time. Not today. Not while I have any influence. And so, I have secretly shot a bigger woman, with big breasts. Not the spherical, hard balloons imposed upon us by surgery and society, but real ones. Pendulous ones. With blue veins. She has bouncy pillows of hair emerging from her bikini bottoms, a sort of modern-day Maria Schneider from Last Tango in Paris. The woman is laughing. Impossibly confident in her skin. The cover line? That, my friends, is my pièce de résistance.

'What Love Island would look like if women ruled the world.'

I was nervous the editor would hate it. Throw me out for crimes against fashion.

She had picked up the photo, propped it up against her computer. 'Wow,' she said. 'This is brave. Might get me sacked but – you know what? – these days, they wouldn't dare.'

She called in the features editor, who was slightly annoyed, tbh, to be dragged away from scrolling houses on Rightmove, and showed her my cover. The woman

266

looked scared but, seeing her boss's enthusiasm, tried to act supportive.

'But what on earth will go inside?' she'd asked us. 'The photo is all very well. But what about my section of spa reviews? There's no time to commission anything else. I'm going on holiday and then I've got maternity leave.'

I told them not to panic, Mr Mainwaring. That I'd already written a piece. About my tummy tuck. The lipo. The pain. The screaming while burping. The gay husband. The new boyfriend who left me for someone not even thinner, but certainly dimmer. The editor looked thrilled. (Wow, this woman is a complete ghoul.) 'Any photos of all the surgery?' she'd said, ever the professional. They always want more. They always want blood.

'Yes,' I said, placing two piles on the desk: one the befores, the other the afters, taken by the fatigue wearing nurse-sniffer. 'Here they are. Have them. I no longer care. I have nothing to hide. The copy is already in your in box.'

. . .

I went to pick Mum up on the 23rd and as I parked the Polo outside the door of the sheltered housing complex, I caught sight of her, unguarded, in her sitting room. It was as though I was seeing her for the very first time. She was already in her wheelchair, with her coat on, tinsel in her hair, a pile of presents piled precariously in her ample lap, as well as a fast defrosting Butterball turkey and an expectant look on her large, shiny face. She kept glancing at her watch and craning her neck. And I knew, I just knew with every fibre of my being, that I would not be able to bring myself to return her to this place. She belongs with us. Not strangers. I will tell her my plan tonight, once we've eaten and she has a schooner of Harvey's Bristol Cream inside her; the twins are fit to bursting with holding in the secret. I had discussed it with them first, of course, as it will mean a big change for them. They didn't hesitate. They even offered up their bedroom, until I explained she can no longer do stairs.

She will worry and say what about her things, and meeting new carers, as she's become quite fond of her current ones, and what about if I decide to take my husband back ¬— I haven't yet broken it to her he's gay. She will meet his new boyfriend tomorrow; if she starts to express astonishment, I will simply shove a sprout in her mouth – but I will just have to be gently persuasive. I will tell her I will go and pack up all her stuff in the New Year. That she no longer has to worry 'bout a thing.

This afternoon, Neps!, calling round to drop off the twins' presents, also brought a huge veggie curry his mum had made us. It's been amazing how everyone has rallied round. Even the neighbours whose names I can never remember brought a cake. He was giving me detailed instructions on what to do with the curry, so I told him my plan for Mum. To my huge surprise, he offered to help me with a van to collect all her stuff, her lovely stuff, and I find I just cannot wait; I didn't have to ask, or ask again, or plead, or nag, or email him, or squawk 'Neps!', 'Neps!', 'Neps!'. It's a bleeding Christmas miracle.

With my new workload and no husband around all the time (he's no longer contesting that I get to keep the house; he has also agreed to help pay for the twins, offering far more than is required by law), I realise I must have someone there for when they get home, school holidays and work trips. But it's not just that. I am not that insanely selfish. I'm beginning to realise, too, that surely the role of a woman is not to be a sex kitten, or a slave to our kids, or a workaholic, or a long-suffering wife, or an interior decorator, or a self-hater, or a cleaner, or an expert in self-denial, or an Olympic gymnast, or Sisyphus, but to be a proper daughter to the woman who squeezed us out from between her ample thighs.

And so it is, on Christmas Eve, I'm on the saggy sofa in my saggy trackie bottoms on my still slightly saggy arse, with the twins, Mum and Izzy, who has escaped the clutches of her family for once. 'I thought Muslims weren't allowed to drink,' my mum said at one point, all innocence, as Izzy lined up the glasses.

'I'm lapsed,' she'd said, laughing, popping open another bottle. I went over and hugged her. I'd been to her family home once, shocked at how she opened the door wearing a headscarf, at how subservient she'd seemed. I know she can never, ever take a man of her own choosing home to meet her father. Even though she has her own business, they never shower her with praise, only disapproval. We all have our problems. Some of us just moan more loudly. In future, I'm trying to be more grateful for what I do have. I am going to be a better friend. A better daughter. I don't need a man to complete me.

It's now nearly midnight, and we're all wearing Christmassy onesies, given we all had to undo our trousers after the curry. The twins have draped silver rain atop Mum's head and we are ready for bed, eating great big bowls of ice cream. The full-fat stuff. None of your frozen yogurt nonsense. All the prep for lunch tomorrow is done; I've even invited Neps! and the Ginger Beard, which is the moment I've chosen to break the news to Mum he's gay. The twins already know, I think. 'Dad is really into fashion,' I heard them tell a little friend we were ferrying to swimming.

I am not inviting Jeremy and Deidre, though: I have my limits. I haven't even clapped eyes on him. Occasionally, in an idle moment, I will search Amazon for the latest bestsellers, but his name is never on the list. Good. Serves him right. You see, I wasn't holding him back from a wonderful career after all. He was just making excuses. I sometimes wonder if they are still together and I occasionally look up her Facebook page, thwarted when there are no clues. It seems she is still in New York, though, so the move can't have happened. Maybe in saving myself, I saved her, too.

Mum has been marinating her turkey all day. It is now crouched in the garden, as it's too big for the fridge, and the cat keeps eyeing it; he is on the back of the sofa, making a long sausage, a small twitch at the end of his tail betraying his anger at the cat flap being locked. It's A Wonderful Life is playing on Channel 5 and we are now at the bit where James Stewart returns home to his family, to find his house is not a leaky, abandoned wreck, but a warm, twinkly home. His wife is not a bespectacled old maid, working in a library. He is no longer bankrupt and headed for jail and his children wonderfully, beautifully exist. He hugs them to him with his great big hands and the tears fall from my eyes and down my shiny face as I hug my little ones, as soft as pillows, close. How different our lives would be, if we only made different choices. Because everything is a choice. I chose to mainline Walnut Whips. No one forced me.

After the curry and the clearing up, I tell the twins

to line up and stand up straight and get ready to hug Granny; they are so excited, as they know what I am about to say. They are actually shaking and hopping. Izzy, who is so happy to be here as part of my unusual little family, especially as we have champagne on tap, unfolds her iPad and starts to film us, trying not to shake as she is sobbing, too.

'Mum,' I say with as much gravitas as I can muster. She looks up from burrowing in the hippo-sized tin of Quality Street, emerging to brandish one of the horrid strawberry jelly ones triumphantly. 'Yes, dear?' she says, unwrapping the sweet, popping it in her mouth, washing it down with Harvey's Bristol Cream. 'Look, I've found you a purple one, the one with a hazelnut.'

I take the sweet from her, place it carefully to one side.

'Mum. Concentrate. Focus. Stop chewing. Swallow. Me and the twins have got something really, really important we want to ask you …'

The End

POSTSCRIPT
(and an admission)

Helen Fielding wrote recently that she has never eaten more than 30,000 calories in one day, nor been unsure of the paternity of her unborn child, but that Bridget Jones was of course based on her. While best friend Shazzer was based on her friend in real life, Sharon Maguire.

I too have never been over a size 18 (I doubt I've ever been above a size 10; actually, if I am ever over an 8, I still go into a bit of a decline), had a tummy tuck or liposuction, owned a pitta bread flap of skin or been married to a gay man (I did, once, live in Brixton, though). I don't store cheese pasties in my handbag. But I have to admit here that both Big Pam and Little Pam are based on real people.

Little Pam is basically me. I am your typical skinny, self-obsessed, no-pudding-for-me-thanks-very-much-I'm-really-full stick insect, OCD-to-a-David Beckham-level nightmare.

I wrote this novel because I have wasted my entire life trying to be something I am not and I would hate for any

273

other woman to waste her life in the same way. I have always been slim, but never quite thin enough if the pages of Vogue are to be believed. I have always thought my life will begin … when I'm down to my target weight (the clue is in the title of this book), or have bought that Alexander McQueen jacket (or, in fashion parlance, 'runway look') with the lace hem costing £4,000, or when my house has been spring-cleaned (dear God, to own a house! I lost mine when I was made bankrupt in 2017; that's a whole other book), or I've been freshly extreme bikini waxed, or my lashes and brows and hairline freshly inked. Or when I have just been spray-tanned in a little cubicle: you see, I even wanted to belong to a different ethnicity, so badly did I hate myself, and still do, to some extent. The to-do list is endless before I can really get going and LIVE!, before I am ready to face the day, get a boyfriend, enjoy myself. Oh, and that's another one: like Little Pam, I have that disease where you can never experience happiness. I am permanently sad, like Lucy in Charlie Brown: a manic depressive, if ever I've met one.

Like Big Pam, though (it's a little confusing, so please do try to keep up) I have had plastic surgery: a facelift, accompanied by eye bag removal or, as it is called in the trade, blepharoplasty. It was painful, expensive and I found that being in possession of a new, strange face didn't really change my life, or inspire a man to love me, or make me love myself (it did, though, momentarily confuse my Border Collies, who barked, failing for a moment to recognise me).

Like Big Pam, I woke up from the anaesthetic and wished with every fibre of my being I could be dead because I realised I'd made a stupid mistake, believing if only I looked younger life could start, wishing that the operation had never taken place due to a power cut or the fact the surgeon had to rush home to feed his very hungry cat. I have tried to commit suicide, twice, and while I have been roundly criticised for writing about the desperate times in my life, the conjoined twins that are depression and anxiety and complex post-traumatic stress disorder in my newspaper columns, I believe the fact so many women and men are driven to want to end their lives, who live in so much pain, with no light at the end of the tunnel, means we should write about it, joke about it irreverently much, much more, not less. Just because an issue is out in the open does not encourage others to copy, or wallow. When I became anorexic, aged 11, I never knew that what I was doing had a name. I had never heard of anyone else who tried to starve themselves. I thought I was the first. That I had invented it. That I was unique.

I've never dated a Jeremy and my mum, though she was bedridden for the last ten years of her life, and who was always a little bit fat, and endured the horrible, crippling pain and disfigurement of arthritis, never suffered from MS. My dad didn't run off when I was eight; he stuck around till he was 82. The only time he ever referred to my extreme anorexia was to exclaim one Saturday evening during Dr Who: 'Mummy! Lizzie has no bottom!' My eating disorder meant I was not just too shy to ever meet men in my twenties, meaning I remained a virgin until I was 32, but I never menstruated. Which means I've never given birth to twins, or even ones. Which means, just like Big Pam, I entirely wasted my twenties being unhappy and self-hating, only for slightly different reasons. If you are still that young, take heed. That decade will be over in the blink of an eye. Enjoy yourself. Remember every moment.

But having been a national newspaper columnist for the last 20 years, writing about my own disastrous life and even more disastrous relationships (please don't call me a 'confessional journalist': you would never call a man that, you would just say he is 'honest' and 'brave'), everything else in this book is completely and utterly real. The slights from husbands. The laziness. The cheating. The spousal yoga. The lawnmower Googling. The spousal monosyllabism. The fashion front-row frostiness. The discovery of my husband's emails, professing his undying love for a trollop he met while 'finding himself' in India (where was he, finally? Inside her vagina?). The discovery of incriminating photos on his camera, bought by me at great expense for his trip.

My husband was, and probably still is, an Indian Sikh who had many affairs while we were married and who indeed never did find out how to open the bonnet of the VW Golf I bought him to top up the oil. He didn't leave me for a man. But the serial adultery and the resultant hurt is true.

And pretty much all the dialogue in this book is true, too, overheard during 30 long, Diptyque-scented,

276

staggering-over-cobbles-in-Paris, town car-ferried years at the coal face of innumerable fashion shows and beauty and fragrance and wellness spa launches all over the world (I did to my shame once call reception at a remote spa in Kerala to wail angrily, 'I've forgotten my mantra!'). I did once have the man I love tell me, 'I need to be a dad. And you can't give me that.' A terrible, shattering thing to be told. As if you are not enough. You will never be enough.

So, while Little Pam is basically, unashamedly me, with all her faults and peccadillos, her fear of mirrors and of a man ever seeing her upright, Big Pam is based on two remarkable and very funny women. One, whom I've known for 11 years, a woman who quite often does that begging thing with her hands as paws, usually performed outside the Richmond branch of Greggs, and a friend who works in PR and once introduced me to David Cassidy before he died, for which huge thanks and if I can ever afford to buy a house again, I'm leaving it to you both to share nicely.

The beads of sweat on noses, even in snow, the endless diets, the puffing up again like a Vesta chow mein, the weight management team, the threat of type 2 diabetes, the self-flagellation, the plucking of sweater over buttock shelf, the cushion on the ample lap, the inability to cross their Miss Piggy legs without pinging and putting someone's eye out, the past-its-sell-by-date cheese and onion pasty chomping, the having to be dragged up a hill by a large Labrador while trying to jog with boobs flying in your face: all came from the mouths of these two; that is, when they weren't eating. For which huge thanks, and I promise to take you out for a slap-up meal. Except you are both on diet No 2779, which means you are once again weighing coriander and spinach, training for that charity half marathon (sod cancer victims, I'm just doing this to lose weight!), climbing onto those scales with a heavy (!) heart, taking off all that jewellery, removing those contact lenses, breathing out and gazing, blurrily, optimistic as ever, at the sodding little needle on the dial. Will it be kind to me today? Will it play nice? Or will it break the inevitable, crushing news that I am just not good enough. That I am weak. That I am greedy. That I am sub-standard. That I am a pariah. That I am a drain on the NHS and society in general. That no man will ever love me.

That I am just a little too fat.

Ladies. Just be kind to yourselves.

ALSO BY LIZ JONES

Non-fiction

Slave to the Rhythm:
The Artist Formerly Known as Prince
(Little, Brown, 1997)

Liz Jones's Diary
(Quadrille, 2005)

Fur Babies: Why we Love Cats (Quadrille, 2007)

The Exmoor Files:
How one single girl got married
(Weidenfeld & Nicolson, 2009)

The Girl Least Likely To:

30 years of fashion, fasting and Fleet Street

(Simon & Schuster, 2013)

Printed in Great Britain
by Amazon